CHOOSING WISELY

CHOOSING
WISELY

How Patients and Their Families
Can Make the Right Decisions
About Life and Death

Charles Radey, M.D.

Image Books
DOUBLEDAY

New York London Toronto Sydney Auckland

AN IMAGE BOOK
PUBLISHED BY DOUBLEDAY
a division of Bantam Doubleday Dell Publishing Group, Inc.
666 Fifth Avenue, New York, New York 10103

IMAGE and DOUBLEDAY are trademarks of Doubleday,
a division of Bantam Doubleday Dell Publishing Group, Inc.

LIBRARY OF CONGRESS CATALOGING-IN-PUBLICATION DATA

Radey, Charles.
   Choosing wisely : how patients and their families can make the right decisions about life and death / Charles Radey.
    p.   cm.
   Includes bibliographical references.
   1. Terminal care—Moral and ethical aspects. 2. Death—Moral and ethical aspects. 3. Medical ethics. I. Title.
  R726.R34 1992
  174'.24—dc20   92-10504
                                                      CIP

ISBN 0-385-42463-1
Copyright © 1992 by Charles Radey, M.D.
All Rights Reserved
Printed in the United States of America
October 1992

1 3 5 7 9 10 8 6 4 2

First Edition

For Marcia

The characters in this book are real; the events depicted are true. In order to strictly protect the privacy of patients and their families and the confidentiality of the medical encounter, names, places, and many details have been altered. My aim has been to disguise the external particulars while at the same time preserving the core truth of the stories I have witnessed.

CONTENTS

Introduction		1
Chapter 1:	Informed Consent: The Key to Shared Decisions	7
Chapter 2:	Intensive Care Unit: The Place Between Life and Death	27
Chapter 3:	Critical Care Decisionmaking	40
Chapter 4:	Planning for Illness	93
Chapter 5:	Growing Older: Ethical Issues in Aging	125
Chapter 6:	Tapping Ethics Resources	161
Appendix I:	The Technology of Intensive Care	196
Appendix II:	Designation of Patient Advocate Form	215

Introduction

Medicine has become the modern arena of choice. In the past, war and revolution and tumultuous social change were some of the events that forced men and women to confront difficult choices. In the last half of the twentieth century, medicine, that is, Western medicine, technically driven and efficiently organized, has risen to prominence both as a social phenomenon and as a force in individual lives. Medicine has managed to focus our hopes and dreams as well as our fears and follies on a screen of consciousness. The images are both engrossing and disturbing.

For all its "miracles," for all its efficacious drugs, for all its surgical advances, medicine today seems genuinely confused about its role in society, confused even about its own identity. Computerized scanners and nuclear magnetic imagers produce diagnostic pictures of unparalleled clarity. Yet no instrument exists that can provide insight into the causes of the modern medical malaise.

2
CHOOSING WISELY

Though science and its practically oriented cousin, technology, have delivered a wealth of goods to the practice of medicine, they have at the same time raised public expectations to such a degree that the basic assumptions of our culture have been altered—sickness is unnatural, death is unreal. The common belief is that the precision and predictability of science can be readily translated to our common world of illness, suffering, disability, and death. People expect perfection. For example, nothing but a perfect baby is acceptable. After all, what are amniocentesis, genetic counseling, ultrasound, and fetal surgery for?

With the heightened level of public expectation, the notion of tragedy has almost disappeared from the modern American vocabulary. Instead, an accident, a bad surgical outcome, an imperfect newborn, a postsurgical complication—in short all disappointments and setbacks—are now almost always considered someone's fault. Legal remedies and a flowering language of "rights" have replaced any sense of the fragile, fateful, and vulnerable voyage we are all taking through life. Science will not allow what Shakespeare and Tolstoy knew intuitively: that our lives are not completely our own, that our freedom has boundaries, that terrible fates can befall us, and that ultimately, though tragic at its core, life is a serious and delicious experience.

If we agree that there is no technological fix for the fundamental questions about what life is all about, then where do we turn? The long-run answer perhaps is that we try to draw up as much wisdom as we can from all the deep wells we know. Taking the humanities seriously, reveling in literature, philosophy, art, and history, can in time lead to the sort of reflection that might offer occasional insight into our lives.

But in the short term we all have to struggle in a world of moral ambiguity and uncertainty. We sometimes have to beat on, in F. Scott Fitzgerald's phrase, "boats against the current," trying

INTRODUCTION

to discover what, all things considered, is the best thing to do. Nowhere is this kind of struggle more apparent than in the world of medicine. If rapid change has befuddled practitioners, it has affected patients even more. More and more patients and their families have to come face-to-face with the institutional juggernaut of the modern hospital and are asked to make decisions for which nothing in their past experience has prepared them. Even the medical renditions served up by movies and soap operas cannot prepare a family for the rupture of identity that occurs with illness or the realities of medical treatment in a technobureaucratic environment.

The previous eras of medicine had very few therapeutic options to offer patients. There were few if any interventional technologies to consider, few curative treatments, minimal patient expectations. Now all that has changed as the technological imperative has asserted itself: What can be done must be done. A panoply of choices presents itself to the practitioner and the patient. It is a veritable existentialist's delight! Whereas before the choices were simple and few, now the choices are vexing and many.

This book is about ethics, which is about choices. How best to choose given a specific medical scenario is the crux of the chapters that follow. Notice the book is not about what to choose, or what I would choose, but really about the process of choosing. From my own practice of medicine and later in my fellowship education in bioethics, I have almost daily witnessed the revealing drama of patients and their doctors making decisions. What I remember most is not the drama of diagnosis or the turmoil of a physical or psychological infirmity. It is not even the extraordinary courage of the human spirit in conflict with suffering and death. The drama I'm referring to is the common ground of patients and doctors deciding what to do under difficult circumstances. It is the drama of choice. And it is unfortunately a drama often played out without an adequate understanding of the issues.

Choice is also a prime constituent in the stories of people's lives. To be sure, fate and circumstance play their roles, but the choosing among alternatives is one of the most basic dramas that is imprinted on the human design. Whether to do this or that, chocolate, vanilla, or strawberry, whether to go back to school or not, to accept or spurn a romantic overture, to go on reading this book or not—all of this and more provide a fascinating backdrop for the unfolding stories of our lives. In a way we are the stories of our lives. We live with and in and through stories. Our own story is a river full of unpredictable turns, deep channels, and chancy currents. Human stories have a beginning and an end and a life in the middle riddled with choices. When serious illness taps us on the shoulder and we have to face the unpleasantness of our mortal natures, the choices involved in trying to restore vitality and stave off death are magnified. The daily choices we so unconsciously make are no longer so mundane. In a strange and paradoxical way, illness illuminates the sweet profundity of life. By turning the view of the afflicted inward, sickness becomes the occasion of significant choices in a person's life. These choices in turn create not only the plot but the very texture of the unfinished story of our life. And it is precisely at this point that bioethics can make a contribution.

Although the study of ethics in medical schools and residency programs has significantly increased in the last ten years, doctors in general are not comfortable with addressing ethical issues in patient care. The practical wisdom, deliberation, and reflection needed do not come easily to those trained in the fast-paced, result-oriented world of medicine. For many doctors, but by no means for all, ethics is either something private or something with legal undertones. Still, recent years have seen numerous

INTRODUCTION

books, articles, and conferences that address ethical issues in medicine and nursing. Bioethics is on its way to becoming a respected academic and consultative discipline. But unfortunately its educational efforts are oriented to the needs of the practitioner, not the patient.

The lack of specific materials aimed at informing and empowering patients to engage thorny problems in medical ethics is the major reason I undertook the writing of *Choosing Wisely*. All too often I have seen families floundering about for some direction, some basis for thinking through a loved one's plight.

And as a matter of fact, my own interest in bioethics was perked at the time of my father's debilitating stroke, his hospitalization, and his eventual death. I was staggered not only by the shock and suddenness of his illness, but by the feeling that I did not have the requisite ethical bearings needed to make crucial decisions in his care. There was no one to turn to for advice. We drew strength from pulling together as a family, but still felt stuck in a moral morass. Questions about what my father would have wanted done, questions about the possibility of cardiac arrest, about long-term feeding—these all were things we had thought about before in the abstract but about which we felt somewhat helpless in the real world of a family member's medical crisis.

This book is intended to be helpful to both the believer and the unbeliever, the follower of religion and the skeptic. Many writers and commentators about medical ethics have religious and theological training that serves them well in conceptualizing the multiplicity of conundrums spawned by modern medicine. The great religions themselves have spoken on some of the fundamental problems that so vex medicine. Sacred texts as well as letters, encyclicals, advisories, and position statements on various issues all contribute to the broad and many-voiced conversation in bioethics.

I would argue that these voices are worth listening to for both believer and unbeliever. For the person of faith, the insight of a text, the wisdom of a tradition, or the counsel of a minister may be a decisive factor in the illumination of an ethical problem. Religious faith often trumps the rational arguments of philosophy for the person attempting to make a difficult choice. Faith and reason together form a powerful combination. The deliberation and reflection so necessary in the practical consideration of ethical dilemmas are galvanized by both faith and reason.

For the unbeliever, familiarity with religious texts and the intricacies of religious culture is a broadening experience. The realization that religions take moral questions seriously and think of biomedical ethical issues as not entirely understandable or solvable based on the approach of reason alone is in itself a salutary effect. Combined with the skeptic's zeal for questioning and disdain for shoddy thinking, an openness to the spiritual values of religion can round out the rough edges of the prickly contentions of the pure rationalist. Even for the unbeliever, religion can be a humanizing influence that bears directly on struggles of choice in medicine.

The book in hand may not be the first resource to turn to in the event of a perplexing medical treatment decision. My hope is that *Choosing Wisely* may complement the wisdom and experience of family and friends and serve as a starting point for deeper reflection and study about the rending choices that we all have to face.

CHAPTER 1

Informed Consent: The Key to Shared Decisions

"He had surrendered all reality, all dread and fear, to the doctor beside him, as people do."
—William Faulkner
Light in August

"Illness wounds, diminishes, and compromises our very humanity and places us in a uniquely vulnerable situation in relation to the professed healer."
—Edmund Pellegrino

The nineteenth-century Russian writer Leo Tolstoy wrote a wise and unflinching novella about sickness and death and its effect on the human spirit. *The Death of Ivan Ilyich* tells the story of a middle-class judicial official who falls mortally ill and must depend on the institutions of his time for comfort and support. Ivan Ilyich must look into the heart of suffering in order to discover the meaning of compassion. He must suffer isolation and loneliness in order to find the warmth of the human circle. And finally, he must suffer spiritual desolation in order to find God.

Truly in Tolstoy's story the process of dying comes to life. Tolstoy also creates on the page a feeling for what happens when a person becomes sick and must submit the territory of the flesh

CHOOSING WISELY

to the medical establishment for examination. The sense of terror, bitterness, and powerlessness experienced by Ivan Ilyich in his encounter with doctors has something to teach us more than one hundred years after the story was written.

Early in the novella, after experiencing a strange taste in his mouth and a slight discomfort on his left side, Ivan Ilyich, at his wife's insistence, decides to consult a celebrated physician. This is the first of many transactions with men of medicine in the book:

> The whole procedure was just what he expected, what one always encounters. There was the waiting, the doctor's exaggerated air of importance (so familiar to him since it was the very air he assumed in court), the tapping, the listening, the questions requiring answers that were clearly superfluous since they were foregone conclusions, and the significant look that implied: "Just put yourself in our hands and we'll take care of everything; we know exactly what has to be done—we always use one and the same method for every patient, no matter who." Everything was just as it was in court. The celebrated doctor dealt with him in precisely the manner he dealt with men on trial.
>
> The doctor said: such and such indicates that you have such and such, but if an analysis of such and such does not confirm this, then we have to assume you have such and such. On the other hand, if we assume such and such is the case, then . . . and so on. To Ivan Ilyich only one question mattered: was his condition serious or not? But the doctor ignored this inappropriate question.*

---

* Leo Tolstoy, *The Death of Ivan Ilyich* (New York: Bantam Books, 1981), pp. 74–75.

INFORMED CONSENT: THE KEY TO SHARED DECISIONS

So Ivan Ilyich meets his fellow professional. One is struck by the pretension of their respective roles, which is instantly recognized by Ilyich, the court official. Though we are not privy to the mind of the physician in this case, one wonders if he is blind to his own pretensions, unable to see what the sick and worried court bureaucrat can so clearly see. Does the fact of illness confer an intolerance of the daily airs and puffery that would normally be endured? Here Ilyich must suffer the humiliation of being powerless before a magistrate of medicine. The tables are turned. He does not like the disadvantage and vulnerability of his new position.

Here we come to the lessons of the story. How can each of us as a patient (a role most of us play sooner or later) prepare ourselves so that the feelings of impotence and anger do not spoil the possibilities of healing and care that should be at the center of the patient-doctor relationship. In short, how can you take on more power in the patient role to achieve a counterbalance to the powers of medicine and its large institutions? I think that by more thoroughly understanding the notion of informed consent, you can take a large first step in the direction of greater comfort and shared responsibility for your own health care.

Background

When you think about what happens between doctors and patients, it is really quite remarkable. You agree to turn your body over for close scrutiny, for testing that invades your very flesh. Every abnormal sound or lump or discoloration invites further investigation. For the physician, every bodily orifice is an opportunity. Samples of tissue might be taken for microscopic examination. Powerful X-ray beams and drugs at the physician's suggestion can be loosed on the flesh. And the good doctor, attired in a crisp white lab coat accompanied by a gaggle of assistants in a clean, upscale office with his Mercedes or BMW discreetly parked in back, looks squarely at you (mind you, he's a busy man!) and tells you what he thinks should be done next. Gigantic institutions stand ready behind the doctor willing and able to carry out his plans.

And you are left on the examination table, perhaps not fully clothed, to contemplate what is happening, because it's not exactly clear.

The notion of informed consent is central to every encounter in medicine. Without informed consent a patient blindly presents his or her body to a practitioner to do with what the doctor wills. With the accomplishment of informed consent, the patient participates in the process of decisionmaking with the caregivers. Although the case-law foundations of informed consent are relatively new, the common-law notion of respect for bodily integrity is centuries old. Still, the idea that the patients and physicians should jointly decide treatment issues is resisted by many in the medical profession at the same time it is accepted by an increasingly critical and demanding public. Judge Cardozo's decision in 1914 laid legal groundwork for the informed consent cases later in the century: "Every human being of adult years and sound mind has a right to determine what shall be done with his own body."

Some doctors see the doctrine of informed consent as a threat to professional autonomy. The problem has been the reluctance of physicians to share information. The patient's appetite for information is seen by many doctors as an unjustified intrusion into professional judgment and expertise. The recent consumerism of many patients has blunted the former unquestioned perogatives of the medical profession. More and more patients now demand more and more information from their physicians.

Informed Consent as Shared Decisionmaking

So just what is this beast, informed consent? Basically it is the attempt of the two parties of the medical relationship to come together and share in the decisionmaking process. On the one hand, we have the patient. In illness this means a vulnerable, needy person "ruptured" from the general flow of life, as writer and neurologist Oliver Sacks has noted. For the seriously ill or injured, the future is cut off, hopes are negated, dreams are deferred. At this time of greatest vulnerability and fear, you are asked to make a series of weighty decisions regarding your care.

On the other side of the table is the physician. The physician brings authority, a wealth of information and knowledge about the given disease process afflicting the patient, and an expert sense of how the medical system works. You can readily see how asymmetrical the relationship is between doctor and patient. On the turf of the medical office or the hospital room the preponderance of the power is with the doctor. This lack of balance underscores the responsibility of caregivers to provide information that will equalize the disproportion of power.

This disproportion of power inherent in the medical encounter is sometimes expressed in subtle ways. I am reminded of a technique used by magicians called a "force." When, for example, a member of an audience is asked to select a card from a full deck ("Take a card, any card!") or to choose among objects X, Y, or Z, the magician manipulates the apparent choice such that the participant ends up being able to choose only what the magician wants chosen. This "force" is both a physical and a psychological manipulation.

When I was taking one of my surgery rotations, I observed the same sort of behavior in a surgeon's office. After a patient was examined, tested, and diagnosed with gallbladder disease, he was presented with alternative scenarios. The first choice was to not have surgery but instead to alter the diet and see what develops. The second option was to have surgery and remove the distressed gallbladder, but to postpone the surgery as far into the future as possible. The third option was to have gallbladder surgery as soon as possible. "Get it over with, save yourself a lot of pain and worry," said the surgeon as he completed his "force." Whether it was conscious or unconscious, the surgeon tilted perceptibly toward the option of immediate gallbladder surgery, making it seem the only truly reasonable choice. The patient was manipulated into a position of seeming to freely choose surgery. The asymmetry of power in the relationship was clearly evident. In effect, the surgeon not only had all the cards, but dealt from a stacked deck.

Elements of Informed Consent

For the patient to avoid such disadvantage, the power of knowledge must flow toward him or her. What is the conscientious physician obliged to disclose to you, the patient? The basic rule of disclosure in conversing with a patient about a contemplated treatment is to tell all information that a reasonable person in the same circumstances would find material and necessary to make a decision. These elements are:

INFORMED CONSENT: THE KEY TO SHARED DECISIONS

1. The nature of the test, procedure, treatment, or surgery. The description should be in words you understand—plain English (or Spanish or Vietnamese). Don't let your doctor get away with a lot of medical gobbledygook. If necessary, tell him that you don't understand a given point and that you cannot consent until you do.

2. Risks should be discussed. You should be informed about the probability and magnitude of all risks; your physician may not inform you of remote or very unusual risks unless their utter seriousness demands disclosure. For example, if a procedure entails a slim chance of death, this should be mentioned. On the other hand, if a given procedure has a one-in-a-hundred chance of your breaking out with a minor skin rash, your doctor may not mention this possibility.

    Also, and this is controversial, risks may be hidden from you if in the practitioner's opinion knowledge of the risks will cause you harm. This is known as the doctrine of "therapeutic privilege" and is seldom justifiable since in essence the harm of the truth must be shown to be greater than the harm of lying to a patient.

3. The benefits of the proposed procedure should be discussed. Why should you consent to this proposed procedure? You should know if there is a probability of complete or partial benefit from a treatment. Could this be an experiment or procedure with no direct benefit for you?

4. Are there alternative therapies? What would happen if you postponed a contemplated procedure or surgery or substituted another treatment? Question your practitioner. And then question still more.

    If these issues are discussed over time and without undue haste or pressure, we could confidently say that you have voluntarily consented. Furthermore, the consent is based on the knowledge that has accumulated over the course of time regarding the treatment decision. It is also based on the accrued trust that has developed between you and your doctor as both have engaged in the process of informed consent.

Advantages of Informed Consent

The advantages of this collaborative approach to treatment decisions are mutual. Most important, your autonomy and bodily integrity are respected. For the physician, the process of informed consent allows a kind of disciplined self-scrutiny and shared responsibility for what are in truth daunting demands and duties. Informed consent also promotes a sober assessment of treatment prospects so that puffery, inflated claims, and exaggerated expectations are effectively quashed.

One thing is certain. Informed consent has nothing to do with a delegated nurse rushing up to your bed, form in hand, and asking you to sign a "consent form." No assurance "that it's all just routine" should tempt you to cooperate with such a frivolous nod in the direction of informed consent. *Not* signing such a form without first engaging in the kind of process described above will quickly bring any treatment to a halt. Soon you will be surrounded by practitioners eager to give the information you seek. So don't be buffaloed by pro forma forms. Remember that some very prestigious medical centers dispense with such a form, believing this encourages doctors to obtain and record on the chart a patient consent that resembles the reality of the information given to the patient.

INFORMED CONSENT: THE KEY TO SHARED DECISIONS

The Ethical and the Legal

The American writer and professional cynic Ambrose Bierce in his *Devil's Dictionary* defined the moral as "conforming to a local and mutable standard of right. Having the quality of general expediency." The law takes a more serious and less jaundiced view of what is right behavior.

Before going on to chapters focused on specific ethical questions, it might be well to talk about the relationship of ethics to law. By elucidating some of the differences that these two disciplines bring to solving biomedical problems, I hope to show how both may contribute to our society's conversation about choices.

Law refers to codes, legislative acts, and case precedents that together form a body of legal thought. Though law may make a society function better, that is with some degree of fairness and equity, it is not necessarily the best vehicle for solving complex ethical problems. This is especially true in areas of personal conduct—for example, the rightness or wrongness of premarital sex. The law can operate only at the extremes of this issue, forbidding such fringe behaviors as rape or the sexual abuse of children. The more subtle forms of coupling are rightly out of bounds as far as legalities are concerned but very appropriately the object of ethical consideration. Likewise, in a hospital-treatment decision, beyond defining rough boundaries (battery, murder, and extortion of patients are clearly forbidden), the law must in most instances stand back and let the patient, his or her family, and the caregivers work out complex issues within the boundaries of case precedent and legislative acts.

But because the boundaries of legal concern are not always clear and the point at which ethics and medicine diverge is often murky and indistinct, many problems in medical ethics have ended up before a court of law. *Roe* v. *Wade* and the Karen Quinlan case are well-known instances where the law has spoken on a bioethical matter. Interestingly, these two cases speak to a pair of issues that are truly indistinct at the margins, troubling to a wide spectrum of society, and philosophically unresolvable to everyone's satisfaction. Hence, to decide when life begins and when meaningful life ends, we have tended to turn to the law for an opinion. Often a series of court decisions that describe, modify, or elaborate are rendered about the truly tough problems like abortion and treatment at the end of life. In a way, the recent decision in the Cruzan case, which, if you remember, dealt with a young woman who had been maintained with a feeding tube for more than seven years following an automobile accident and had existed in a comalike limbo called the persistent vegetative state, the Supreme Court of the United States passed down an opinion that built on previous decisions, mostly from various state supreme courts. The court then went on to develop new law concerning the so-called right to die and specifically ruled on the question of whether Nancy Cruzan had left proper advance directives for her care. There will be more cases before many courts that will seek to define more precisely the duty of care and the limits of treatment.

Insofar as courts and legislatures have dealt with medical ethics issues, the inherent tension between a legalistic and an essentially philosophic approach has been all too evident. On very problematical issues there is a lot of buck-passing among legislatures, courts, and the private domain. In a way, Americans seem to need a court decision or a law to build consensus as opposed to building a consensus on a given issue in order to keep the decision out of the legal and legislative worlds.

On the other hand, the European approach to such questions

as abortion has been far less polarized and heated. In many countries of Europe a compromise has been worked out that does not satisfy any contentious party completely but allows society to move on to other business without the paralysis of unending conflict. In other words, a cultural consensus based on compromise has slowly evolved, making reliance on the decision of a high court unnecessary. The danger of relying on a legal decision is that the very terms of debate are reined in and limited to a constitutional or case precedent. The free flow of philosophical, social, and political ideas is not given a full voice as a society wrestles with a difficult issue. Thus our discussion of informed consent has touched many more bases than exclusively legal ones.

Patients, Doctors, and Informed Consent

My experience in clinical medicine has shown me that patients are sometimes tempted to abandon or shirk any idea of sharing responsibility for making decisions. "Whatever you think is best, Doc" or "I'll do whatever you would do, Doc, if you were in my situation" are common responses heard in the office or hospital room. You can gauge your own physician's commitment to the process of informed consent by how he or she reacts to such a statement. If you as a patient (or a relative or friend) attempt to evade or deny sharing responsibility for decisions that will affect your body, does the physician go along with you or does he attempt to give back the power you have inappropriately offered? Physicians who are sensitive to their patients and who see them as free and morally responsive beings will not want to assume the old garb of "doctor always knows best."

CHOOSING WISELY

If we look at just what doctors could possibly know "best," I think you will plainly see that what doctors know best is extremely limited. Doctors know medicine. They know physical diagnosis and treatment of disease. They know lab tests, X-ray studies, and how the latest technology can help in the diagnosis and treatment of illness. Broadly speaking, all doctors know the general process of medicine, for they have all shared a common four years of medical school. Once doctors specialize, as the overwhelming preponderance of medical school graduates now do, they are trained to know more and more about less and less, until at last they are certified as a specialist.

Note that doctors tend to be narrowly trained rather than broadly educated. For many physicians, this narrowing begins in the premed curriculum they choose in college in order to make themselves attractive to a medical school. So unfortunately, medicine is filled with fairly young, technically trained practitioners who have never taken the time to educate themselves in the arts and humanities. Thus, when faced with the vagaries and varieties of human experience in the context of illness, many physicians show little capacity or sensibility to meet the wonders and terrors of the human condition. However, when doctors experience illness themselves, this can open some doors that remain closed to books. A collection of firsthand stories written by physicians, *When Doctors Get Sick,* is very enlightening on this point.*

This usual uncomfortableness with patients can be clearly seen when patients are confronted with a difficult ethical decision. If medical care were merely a technical matter, a doctor could hide behind his technical competence. But when medicine spills over, as it inevitably must, into the broader context of hu-

---

* Harvey Mandell and Howard Spiro, eds., *When Doctors Get Sick,* Plenum Medical Book Company, New York and London, 1987.

man values and the experience of living, the inadequately prepared practitioner is all too oblivious of the patient who seeks to assert moral agency or share a sense of the common human fate. Remember this well: Doctors are not experts about the values you hold that guide and give meaning to your life. And these very values are what will determine the course you follow in a trying situation where choosing the right thing is not easy.

Seeking out the physician with the human touch and the one who has a sense of you as a complete person will be the best assurance that informed consent will be well served. If you feel that conversations with your physician are encounters between equal moral beings who are both trying to do what is right, then you really do not have to worry about whether the specific elements of informed consent are being adequately addressed. Likewise, beware of the doctor who approaches informed consent as a technical or legal burden that he must endure and who would welcome minimal or passive participation from his patients.

Given that doctors are generally overworked and harried, and sometimes sleep-deprived as well, it is no wonder that they yearn for the course of least resistance—the compliant, agreeable patient who readily acquiesces to physician suggestions. Some physicians even feel entitled to patients who will defer to their wishes —given the long, arduous years of study and sacrifice they have made in order to prepare themselves for patient care. As teachers can grow to resent students, and lawyers come to not like certain kinds of clients, doctors, too, can come to positively disdain patients. This paradoxical attitude begins to develop with the excessive patient demands foisted on the doctor during his residency training years. Physicians' wrath and callousness are especially acute toward chronic patients who are seen as self-abusing dregs of the medical system.

If you can recall the realistic portrayal of a large city teaching hospital in the television series *St. Elsewhere,* the program seemed absolutely true to life in its depiction of the haggard interns and their arrogant mentors. But what did not ring true, among other things like excessive violence, was the way in which the young doctors seemed to welcome each new case—the more bizarre, puzzling, and recalcitrant the individual case, the more the resident seemed to like it. This impression runs counter to what I have observed in several different teaching hospitals. In the training environment, patients are a kind of enemy, especially the kind of difficult, down-and-out patients featured on the program. I know it may sound strange to the layperson, but to the fearful, overworked intern or resident, troublesome patients were often seen as the *reason* the young doctor was tired and irritable. Often the ideals of medicine would take a backseat to surviving the rigors of training.

In considering possible barriers to the achievement of informed consent, you must consider where the doctor on the other side of the transaction might be coming from. The foibles and limitations of human nature are magnified in the arena of serious disease and complex choices. It is well to consider the pressures inherent in the doctor role that proceed from the average physician's lack of substantive humanistic education and are nurtured by a medical system that rewards technical competence at the expense of such niceties as informed consent.

Exceptions to the Rule of Informed Consent

There are at least two circumstances where informed consent does not follow the model we have so far developed. The first situation is the medical emergency when consent is presumed due to dire circumstances such as unconsciousness. So if you are involved in an accident and wheeled into an emergency room you will not be expected to spend time establishing informed consent. "Treat first, talk later" is the code of the emergency room in dire cases.

The second exceptional circumstance to consider is if a patient is thought to be incompetent. Is the person capable of making rational decisions, or is this capacity compromised? For the unconscious, permanently vegetative patient, one in the so-called persistent vegetative state (PVS), the conclusion that the patient is unable to make her own decisions is easy. Likewise with persons who are acutely intoxicated or suffering from some sort of metabolic derangement (diabetic coma, for example) or the patient who is grossly retarded or flagrantly psychotic. Though there are no well-accepted standards or rigorous definitions of the state of incompetency, nonetheless the problem is almost always couched in legal or psychiatric terms. The judge or the psychiatrist, with the aid of a hearing and a mental status examination, will ultimately render a competency decision.

It is often the case that a patient is partially competent. This implies that the patient can weigh questions dealing with some aspects of his care and not others that may be too complicated for him to consider. There are also many cases where the patient's state of consciousness waxes and wanes. In the morning, for example, the person considering a medical treatment may be entirely competent to decide important treatment questions; in the evening, given swings in rational functioning due to drugs or darkness or metabolic rhythm, the ability to consent may be significantly impaired. Also how should we think of young adolescents, say children in the thirteen-to-fifteen-year age range? Are they fully or partially competent? Given obvious individual variations, one must take seriously at least the limited capacity of children to make medical decisions.

I remember the case of a fifteen-year-old boy who had undergone several rounds of chemotherapy for his leukemia. When admitted to the hospital for yet another intravenous treatment with drugs that profoundly nauseated and weakened him, the boy loudly and firmly refused any more chemotherapy. This set off reverberations of panic from his nurses to his doctors to his parents. A minister consulted on the case. Then a psychiatrist. Eventually a bioethicist was asked for an opinion in the case.

There was general agreement that the boy was competent and sincere in his treatment refusal. The caregivers agreed to carefully listen to his concerns. Although clearly not an adult, the boy was mature for his years, intelligent, and "hospital smart." Clearly he could not be ignored. No one wanted to tie him to his bed and administer the therapy. After much discussion and cajoling, the boy agreed to a compromise. He would put up with the treatment if he could go home sooner than usual and if new drugs were tried to counter the horrific side effects. The case illustrates that informed consent should be taken seriously even with children and that it may result in more reasoned treatment.

How does a family member or friend proceed when a loved one is hospitalized and either acutely or chronically unable to make decisions? In this situation the surrogate decisionmaker has a large role to play. A spouse, son, daughter, sister, brother or other blood relative, or good friend all are potential surrogates, or persons able to stand in the place of the incompetent patient. There is much more to say about surrogacy, living wills, and advance directives—matters we shall address in Chapter 4.

INFORMED CONSENT: THE KEY TO SHARED DECISIONS

Exercising the Right to Be Wrong

As a patient, you have a perfect right to be wrong. Sometimes physicians and other caregivers are all for informed consent as long as the patient chooses the option that they would have chosen. But if a choice runs counter to the values and experience of the physician, it is often questioned. Often a psychiatric evaluation will be requested if the patient's choice is too anomalous or weird. (But conversely, no one would ever think of ordering a psychiatric evaluation of a patient who agreed, for example, to a radical new surgery that had little chance of success. Likewise the sanity of the surgeon who suggests such an operation is never questioned.) Often family members will be enlisted to persuade or badger recalcitrant patients who refuse to consent to a given procedure. Seldom if ever will your competence be questioned if you are agreeable and compliant with the medical authority who has enlisted the confidence of your family members.

I remember Evelyn Weaver, a small-framed, gentle woman in her mid-seventies who began to experience episodes of chest pain. They bothered her most when she was making beds or climbing stairs. She described the pains to me and said it was as if two giant hands were grabbing her heart and twisting it like wringing the water out of a dishrag. The pains stopped her in her tracks and brought this otherwise healthy woman in to see her physician. For a year or so, progressive medical therapy with drugs helped Mrs. Weaver's heart. The therapy allowed more oxygen-rich blood to nourish her heart. For a while she resumed her household activities, but as time went on, even with full medical therapy she began to experience the fearsome chest pains again.

Mrs. Weaver was referred to a cardiologist, who after extensive tests in turn referred her to a cardiac surgeon. The surgeon believed Mrs. Weaver would be a good candidate for cardiac bypass surgery, a procedure that would in effect create a new blood vessel to replace a main vessel in her heart that was ninety-five percent blocked. At seventy-four years of age, the thought of open heart surgery gave Mrs. Weaver and her family pause. They started to pursue information about the risks and benefits of such a procedure. They talked to their family physician, to friends, to the cardiologist, and to the cardiac surgeon. They puzzled over the question of whether to risk the surgery or to risk continuing drug therapy.

Then one day Mrs. Weaver experienced chest pain that just would not go away. Even after three nitro tabs under her tongue, the crushing, squeezing pain persisted. Her husband rushed her to the hospital. By this time she was barely conscious, sweaty, and very weak. The diagnosis of heart attack was evident to the emergency room physician who instituted lifesaving procedures to stabilize her heart rhythm and blood pressure. After three days in the hospital it was evident from her cardiac studies that Evelyn Weaver had been lucky. The heart attack had been a mild one. Suddenly the decision of whether to have surgery was clarified. Evelyn Weaver at age seventy-four with a failing heart was surrounded by risks. To live on, with or without surgery, would be extremely risky.

The family was galvanized to make a decision. They talked among themselves, a husband almost paralyzed with the prospect of losing his partner, and the four adult children who realized their mother was in big trouble. Within weeks of her heart attack Evelyn Weaver underwent successful bypass surgery. She died eight weeks later of massive complications following her surgery, including a stroke, a wound infection in her chest, and a pulmonary embolus. She never left the cardiac intensive care unit after

INFORMED CONSENT: THE KEY TO SHARED DECISIONS

her surgery. She never regained full consciousness. She suffered greatly the assault of respirators, central blood lines, and tube feedings.

Her family suffered with her. Not only did they have to watch what Evelyn endured postsurgically, but all of them were terribly distraught about persuading her to have the surgery done. They could not imagine or foresee the horrors that befell her. They felt they had done everything right in learning about the risks and benefits of the proposed operation. All their hopes and plans for surmounting the illness had come to something less than zero. They were all sorry they had chosen to go through with the surgery. They felt their loved one's fate following surgery was a fate worse than death—a circumstance that they had failed to calculate in their presurgery deliberations.

You can easily feel the pain of the Weaver family. I think this case illustrates that life is far more complicated than medical science or human foresight can anticipate. Sometimes things don't work out for the best. Some decisions will inevitably turn out to be wrong. Even with the best of informed consent, the body can fail unpredictably. What we are left with in this case is some inkling of the tragic dimension of the lives we are living.

Garrison Keillor once told a story on his Saturday night radio program about an old man in a nursing home who one night unexpectedly exercised his personal autonomy and made a momentous decision. The gentleman had been involved in some serious thought throughout the afternoon. Then it was dinnertime. The staff was serving mashed potatoes, and when they came to this old man, he seemed a bit taken back as if his thought processes had been interrupted. He said, "Thanks, no more for me." As other dishes passed the old man, he repeated, "Thanks, no more for me." Well, you haven't had any yet. You've got to eat, they said. You usually like the food, they pointed out. He answered reasonably, "It's not the potatoes or the peas. They look fine, as always. I mean, I don't want to go on living. I've had my fill of life. It's been good. Thanks, no more for me."

Of course, this kind of expression would lead to great consternation in most hospitals and nursing homes. Still, Keillor's little tale captures a kernel of truth. People can make improbable choices, wrong-headed decisions, and yet continue to be competent moral agents. Perhaps the withdrawing of consent for continuing treatment is but a small visible part of a larger withdrawal —the taking of leave, consciously or unconsciously, from life itself. This humorous vignette demonstrates that for a life to be lived, a person must make daily affirmation that his life is worth living and consent to do what is necessary to maintain life. In short, one chooses to live. When something clicks off, like for the man in Keillor's story, people tend to wither and die.

Remember, you deserve respect for the core ethical quality we all possess which is personal autonomy. Moreover, this respect is part of the larger respect we cultivate for the moral lives of other persons. This appreciation for the deep values of another makes possible relating to that person as a moral peer.

Informed consent begins and ends with the idea that patients and doctors are moral equals. The working out of this equality in ongoing conversation and in the conscious sharing of information is the real test of the notion of informed consent. The tendency of the medical profession in the past to favor discretion and silence over disclosure and conversation has led to mutual distrust. Overcoming this legacy of suspicion must involve both an opening up by physicians and a patient mind-set marked by a skepticism and caution.

CHAPTER 2

ICU: The Place Between Life and Death

"Carts wheel past spread with father, wife, or son at the end of tubing."

—Margi Berger
"Anniversary"

The typical intensive care unit brims over with the latest medical technology. If you were to face a crisis in the ICU, a crisis involving a treatment decision, the least problematical part of your dilemma would be the technology itself. Technology has an answer. Its province is action; its direction is remedy oriented. It fixes problems. The fix works or it doesn't. If it works, the problem is solved. If it doesn't, back to the drawing board. The engineering model, however, tends to break down when ambiguity, doubt, or death draw near and when it is not clear whether the technology is contributing to the alleviation of suffering or to a prolongation of misery. This is a time suited for self-questioning, reflection, deliberation, and soul-searching. This is the domain of ethics.

It was H. L. Mencken who observed that for every problem there is a solution—neat, simple, and wrong. In the intensive care unit, most staff members are acutely aware of the wrenching decisions that patients and family must make. They realize that there is no quick fix, no easy answer for the treatment decisions they are asked to make. But clearly these decisions are not merely medical in nature. Even if they were, they are too important to be left to the medical profession. It is extremely important that patients and family always remember the field upon which ethical problems are decided. This is the field of values—personal, religious, and philosophical—which all people hold in some way, and which guide decisionmaking. It is true that medicine occupies some space on this field of values, but certainly medicine is in no position to dominate the making of value-laden decisions for sick patients.

Andrew's Story

Sometimes the struggle to decide whether to live or whether to die is especially poignant. Sometimes a particular patient is completely lucid about the bad hand the fates have dealt. Or a patient may possess a talent to convey what it is like to inhabit a state of being that is, to the observer's eye at least, not completely the world of the living or of the dead. The question of how far to go with a succession of medical treatments often becomes a question of spiritual as well as physical endurance.

Andrew Simmons is animated and intense in conversation, both bright and insightful about his disease. A young man of twenty-three years, Andrew had the bad luck to inherit a condition which occurs, in varying degrees, about once in every three thousand births—neurofibromatosis, also known as Von Recklinghausen's disease, and more popularly as elephant man's disease. Though born with a genetic predispositon, the disease did not come to the attention of his family or physician until he was thirteen years old. Then the lumpy, noncancerous (though hardly benign) tumors started to appear on his back and chest. Soon he was off to the care of specialists with numerous tests and surgeries to remove the disfiguring growths that were close to the surface of the skin.

Throughout his teenage years Andrew led a close to normal life. No tumors invaded his face or neck, and he resisted any invasion of his natural exuberance for friends, sports, and books. After graduating from high school he continued his academic studies at the University of Washington in Seattle.

But the tumors kept appearing. On one of his numerous CAT scans a worrisome tumor was seen to be invading his spinal cord. Andrew soon had trouble controlling his legs. He found it difficult to walk to classes. The pains in his legs and back started to become more intense. At this point Andrew was forced to acknowledge the inevitably progressive and debilitating quality of his disease. Though the tumors near the skin could be controlled, the internal tumors were beginning to wreak havoc on the interior structures of his body. The more the disease asserted itself, the less Andrew was able to control his life.

After two years of a challenging prepharmacy curriculum, Andrew was forced to withdraw. Not only were his legs useless, but new problems had developed with the spread of the tumors. New growths were infiltrating the delicate mechanisms of the inner ears. Inoperable, the tumors soon caused hearing to be added to his personal casualty list. Andrew Simmons found himself at age twenty both deaf and wheelchair bound.

His parents lavished care and encouragement. They had the financial means to buy the best in treatment and physical rehabilitation services, including the installation of an indoor swimming pool in their home. The whole family, including his two younger sisters, learned American Sign Language. Andrew continued to read avidly and took up the new challenge of watercolor painting.

Because of the proximity of some of his internal tumors to his brain stem, sometimes Andrew would have periods of apnea—he would momentarily stop breathing. Most often he would spontaneously restart. But on one occasion he didn't. His mother, who happened to be in the same room, alertly applied emergency resuscitation. Andrew was brought back to the world of the living from the edge of death.

The next day Andrew confronted his mother. With the precocious wisdom of one who had traveled far in a short time, he looked at his mother, and what he said was not so much a demand or a plea, but more like the sharing of a secret: "Mother, you must not bring me back again."

As time passed, the casualty list of potentialities and powers continued to mount. Vision in the right eye vanished after a tumor impinged on the optic nerve. The left eye was reduced to reading large letters held within twelve inches of the face. Swallowing became a problem. And then swallowing was impossible due again to the encroachment of the tumors.

Andrew would occasionally become weak and incoherent due to insufficient nutrition and hydration. His parents would become frantic with worry and wondered about the medical necessity of a feeding tube. With the intrusion of the tumors into his larynx and the resulting surgery, Andrew permanently lost the voice that once had startled his teachers with its clarity and sensitivity and his parents with its honesty and strength.

The doctors finally recommended that a permanent feeding tube be inserted into Andrew's stomach. He was ambivalent about the idea. He knew he wanted to live, but wasn't sure he wanted to live bound to the tube. He vacillated. He stalled. His periods of incoherence and confusion came more often. Finally, on one particular occasion, the biochemical derangements were too much to bear for his parents. They had to give sustenance to their son of twenty-one years who had lapsed into a semi-con-

ICU: THE PLACE BETWEEN LIFE AND DEATH

scious state. The parents consented to the placing of a temporary feeding tube. It was done.

Andrew resumed his life at home, deaf, half blind, voiceless, wheelchair-bound, and tubed. But he was still determined to maintain as much of his previous activities as possible. Though forbidden by his doctors to swim due to the risk of getting water into his tracheostomy, Andrew did not always take his physician's advice. He was determined to preserve as much muscle tone as possible and got great delight from splashing in the water.

One day Andrew's mother found his wheelchair empty. It was a Wednesday, so Margaret, the woman who helped four days a week with Andrew's care and physical therapy, was not in the house. Mrs. Simmons heard a noise in the swimming pool room. She remembered the doctor's warning about possibly aspirating the chlorinated water directly into the lungs and causing a horrific pneumonia. As she approached the pool, Mrs. Simmons was filled with foreboding. She heard no sounds coming from the water. In the pool she found her son. He was joyously and silently floating on his back in the medium which seemed to soak through his limited body and into his very soul.

Andrew had taped an extension onto his tracheostomy tube to prevent water getting into his lungs. He had then crawled from his room and into the pool. Andrew's mother would always remember the radiance of that moment and marvel at the part of her son that had not been taken away.

The shrunken world of Andrew Simmons became even smaller when he lost the ability to use his arms. Painting, pointing, gesturing, signing, holding hands, all became impossible to do. The back and leg pains were becoming more and more intense and unsettling.

It was at this time that Andrew first asked his father, then his mother, if they would do him the favor of mercifully killing him. He asked to be shot or overdosed with drugs. He explained that his shriveled world contained no more plans, no more hopes, no more dreams, no more ambitions, no more future. He felt frozen in space and time. He told his mother that he felt alive only above his neck.

Andrew was admitted to a major referral hospital to evaluate the latest surgical and pharmacological means of alleviating his fearsome leg and back pain. It was at this time he brought up once again the issue of the feeding tube. Well nourished and completely in command of his faculties, no one could now raise the bugaboo of deranged mentation brought about by an imbalance of nutritional elements. He was competent to make his own decisions. And he aimed to squarely face the issue with his parents and caregivers.

As the disease progressed, Andrew and his family devised an elaborate communication system. As deafness, blindness, and immobility all tried to quash communication, the family deftly countered each new roadblock. Andrew could understand sign language if the signing person was within one to two feet of his left eye. To respond, he would nod when large letters on a plasticized alphabet board were touched. First he would nod when the letter for a word he wished to use was in the correct row indicated by his mother or father, who held the letter chart close to his face at the side of the bed. Then he would nod when the finger going down the row of letters came to the exact letter he wanted to form a word. In this manner he laboriously and determinedly "spoke" in short, frustrating sentences which often wore him out in the work of their construction.

Andrew could also move his left arm slightly. To this arm his parents had attached a string of three or four small bells—the kind often used for Christmas decorations. The bells were rung to get attention, to start a sentence, and to indicate spaces between words when he was spelling out by nodding to the alphabet

ICU: THE PLACE BETWEEN LIFE AND DEATH

chart. Thus vigorous ringing followed by a nod to R and then to U and then to B followed by a short ring; and so on with affirmative nods in turn to L, and to E, and to G and S. And then came the sweet relief of his mother's practiced kneading of the wasted flesh of his legs.

I first met Andrew during his hospitalization for evaluation of pain. His primary physicians had asked for a bioethics opinion regarding his apparent determination to discontinue tube feedings. Andrew's mother explained through sign language that I was a doctor there for a different reason than all her other physicians. This doctor, the mother signed, wants to talk to you about what you want for your treatment. He wants to know if you really want to stop your tube feedings. This is an ethics doctor, the signing said. I wondered if he comprehended, indeed if I comprehended, the meaning of the term "ethics doctor."

Suddenly his mother signed: "Do you want to die?"

The question appeared to momentarily stun Andrew with its bluntness, its bald publicness. It was like bursting into a private room filled with the soul's secrets. He sensed the stranger in the audience around the bedside. His mother repeated the question. Andrew rang his bell emphatically before the last sign had left his mother's hands. He understood the question. It really was quite simple. Did he want to live or did he want to die?

Andrew is now eager for the alphabet chart. He has thought about the question before. He knows in his bones about living and dying and all the stops between. Is this truly what I see in his left eye, in the set of his face?

He nods to D, yes to O and N and then to T followed by the tinkling bell. Then his eyes rapidly follow his father's finger on the chart as he comes to the third vertical row of letters. Yes to K; yes to N; and so with O and W.

All this and he doesn't know! His repeated pleas to die, his rational analysis of his own suffering, his calls to stop the feeding tube—do all these anguished signs mask a profound ambivalence? In the end would he prefer to live in his diminished young body than die? Is there something about his truncated life that magnifies small beams of light into a still-powerful life force?

Andrew now appears agitated. He rolls his head from side to side on the pillow. The right side of his face is swollen, cutting off most light to his right eye. His left eye has the anxious cast of an animal pinned and helpless on a veterinarian's table. His mother says he is angry and flustered. He wrests his left hand free from his mother's and rings the string of bells. He wants to say more.

The glowing good eye rapidly courses the alphabet chart. Andrew chooses an *L*, then an *E*, then a *T*. A single ring. Then an *M*, quickly to *E*. Ring! He is increasingly animated as he goes to *P*, to *R*, to *E*, and back to *P*. He pauses as if lost in the word. He then presses on to *A* and to *R* and to *E* before the word-ending tinkle of the bell. Small droplets of sweat gather on his forehead. He is exhausted. His effort to say has the room completely still.

I think I know what's coming and I say to myself, No, let *me* prepare.

Mrs. Simmons's finger patiently courses the chart. Andrew selects *T* and then *O* before ringing his bell. My eye, his mother's and father's eyes, and Andrew's one good eye all meet at the letter *D* on the chart. He nods. We go on. He chooses *I* and then *E* and his choices resound in the antiseptic space of the hospital room.

No one speaks. Though the telling was hard, Andrew's eye is suffused with a placid gaze. The animal intensity is gone. The pinned and caged part of himself now has plans.

Eventually Andrew consented to have one more neurosurgical procedure that would attempt to disconnect the pain fibers between his legs and back and his brain. The operation was successful. Andrew decided to live on, each day in its own way a preparation for a death that would for him come sooner rather than later.

This Place of Pain and Healing

The intensive care unit, then, is the physical space where the technological wonders of the last twenty years collide with the eternal questions of right and wrong. For the hospital administrator, ICU stands for "intensive cash unit" since each bed is capable of generating thousands of dollars a day for the institution. For the patient, ICU stands for the "intrusive care unit," such are the extent and depth of its psychic and physiological control of its occupants. In this charged environment of serious illness, whole families are stressed to the point of crisis. It is here that grandmother, father, or uncle is plunged into the alien world of monitors and tubes, and the contending voices of hope and despair. It is a disorienting experience to say the least.

Despite the obvious serious nature of intensive care, seventy to eighty percent of ICU patients survive the experience. So there is some reason for optimism in the statistical sense. These units do indeed provide lifesaving care for seriously ill and injured persons.

But a cautionary note about optimism in the ICU. Quite naturally, no one likes being the bearer of bad news, doctors included. Family members, more than the afflicted patient, tend to grab ahold and even magnify any bit of good news from the medical team. Even the slightest report of an improvement in a lab value or an X-ray finding can be the doctor's "gift" to a family eager to hear good news about a loved one. Sometimes the physician's language is filled with medical jargon that a family is unprepared to challenge or even ask for clarification. If the medical intensive care specialist, or simply "intensivist," tells a family member that he is encouraged by their mother's rising cardiac output and falling blood urea nitrogen, further explanation is needed for the typical son or daughter who thinks their mother looks like death warmed over despite the news about cardiac output and nitrogen.

Doctors can be too upbeat because they fear becoming powerless and failing their patient. And like everyone else, at some level they fear death. So though everyone wants to hear good news, we must guard against overoptimistic assessments that in the long run do not improve patient care or add to the chances of making prudent treatment decisions.

"Doctor, Do Everything Possible."

The care of patients threatened with death is fraught with both physical and emotional perils. The challenge of maintaining physiological functioning is a very technical problem for which doctors and other medical personnel are well equipped to handle. The emotional trauma for the patient and family, as well as the caregivers, is something else altogether.

Often a family member of a critically ill or unconscious patient will seek out a physician to let him or her know that they wish their loved one to receive the maximum care level possible. Sometimes a doctor will approach family members with a treatment decision that will in effect gauge the tenor of aggressiveness for a particular patient. The physician is really asking how far do you want us to go in treating Uncle Albert. This is an extremely difficult question to answer!

ICU: THE PLACE BETWEEN LIFE AND DEATH

But the question, no matter what its intent, is often heard by family members as "Do you love your very sick relative?" So the answer to the caregivers is often a reflexive rather than a reflective response. Out of love and to avoid guilt, the reply comes back: "We all love Uncle Albert. Of course we want you to do everything to save his life." Thus starts the long dark night of treatment for many ICU patients.

I would like to suggest that the question is not a technical one, that what *can* be done in the medical sense should not necessarily *be* done. It really is a question of what is appropriate to be done under the specific circumstances of the case. If Uncle Albert cannot speak for himself or has not left advance directives regarding his care, then family members should seek to fathom his mind and past experience and speak faithfully in his place. I can tell you that very few patients choose to live on life support systems. I can think of only one case in my experience where a patient said, yes, I would prefer to live with all these tubes and technology and *never* leave the hospital than not live any longer at all.

The few who do opt for life at any cost or life preserved under any circumstance whatsoever set up biological life as a kind of idol. They generally recognize no possibility of values that go beyond the life of the body. They often do not fairly consider the effects on their living relatives, or caregivers, in their persistent denial of the inevitability of death. And naturally, and how can we blame them, outright primordial fear of death can play a more significant role in some patients as opposed to others. Be aware that there is no argument to be made against this guttural fear. But it must at least be acknowledged if the well are to understand the mortally ill.

The role of physicians in providing maximum life-sustaining care to their patients is somewhat paradoxical. Informal talk in the doctor's lounge, in the hospital corridor, or during a break at a medical conference reveals that on a personal level physicians are repelled by the utter invasiveness of ICU care. They almost always say that they would not want to die this way or live the truncated life of a person on a life support system. Often the joke is heard among medical personnel that they would want the words "do not resuscitate" or "no code" tattooed to their chests lest they fall into the hands of an overly aggressive doctor in an emergency. You might say that physicians fear their own death less than they fear doing less than everything for their patient.

The paradox is that despite their personal thoughts on the subject, physicians will proceed at full speed ahead and pursue every avenue they know to stave off death. Often this is done even in the face of some expressed doubt on the part of the patient or family. Why this contradiction? Why one set of rules for themselves and another for patients?

The answer, I think, lies in a deep desire not to fail the patient. Since the most fundamental level of failing the patient occurs at the physical level, doctors often become trapped in the consideration of preserving organ systems and hence of saving biological life. The ethical and social ramifications of a decision to go all out to save an organ system are of secondary importance to defending the notion that the baseline integrity of what it means to be a physician is exclusively in the physical realm. This fundamentally limited view of the human is evident when doctors speak about the heart or kidney they have helped to save and which now functions inside the intensively cared for patient. Meanwhile visitors see that the whole organism dims as if some inner light has gone out. The patient is saved to "live" another day. The human being is somewhere lost.

Like patients and families, doctors are often perplexed and afraid of the awesome choices that are generated by medicine today. It is obvious that the question of what is appropriate to do in the given circumstances of a case should not be turned over to doctors alone to decide. They are certainly no more morally adept or philosophically informed than the collective wisdom of the patient and family. For truly these kinds of painful treatment decisions tear at the human capacity and inclination to do the right thing. Since doing everything possible often means concentrating exclusively on physiological functioning, and tends to ignore the emotional, the intellectual, and the value aspects of a person, a certain refocusing is necessary. Who is this sick person? What does he stand for? How has he lived his life? These questions and others can point the way toward making appropriate treatment decisions.

The following chapter is meant to home in on specific issues in critical-care medicine. Again I would emphasize that the answer to specific dilemmas of care is not to be found there or anywhere else in this book. My aim is to give a tour of the ethical landscape of the ICU, noting pitfalls, blind alleys, and fruitful paths. My hope is that readers will add to their personal map of the territory of ethics, a map that certainly did not start with this book, but one that has been accruing signs, routes, and directions over the course of a lifetime. The value of a guided tour is an increased ability to ask the right question at the right time. This is *the* crucial skill in facing bioethical problems. Let me repeat this key point: The ability to ask the fitting question at the right time in the midst of a medical/ethical crisis is absolutely essential to arriving at a prudent and informed resolution. The following chapter is designed to aid in the formulation of such questions.

CHAPTER 3

Critical Care Decisionmaking

"Where is the wisdom we have lost in knowledge?
Where is the knowledge we have lost in information?"
—T. S. Eliot

Doris MacSorley is a middle-school teacher who at age forty-four discovered a lump in her right breast. After some months of denial and postponement, she finally consulted her physician. After examining the breast and ordering a mammogram, Mrs. MacSorley was referred to a surgeon. The biopsy turned out to be grim. An aggressive, incurable cancer of the right breast that had already metastasized to her bones. Doris MacSorley was advised to think of her remaining life span in terms of months, five to eight her doctors said.

Since no cure was possible, the medical team concentrated on the patient's comfort. Increasing pain in the right shoulder made each day a trial. The primary care physician referred her to a neurosurgeon, who recommended a rhizotomy—a palliative procedure whereby the spinal nerves to the right shoulder would be severed in order to provide definitive pain relief. Mrs. MacSorley was eager for relief from a pain that was literally taking over her last days and readily agreed to the operation.

The relatively brief surgery went well. But just as the anesthesiologist was preparing to bring her back to consciousness, her heart suddenly went into a dysrhythmia. The electrical impulses that normally set off the heart muscle in a controlled and regular fashion were now completely disorganized. Her heart was no longer pumping blood.

Quick work by the operating room team reestablished an effective heartbeat. Mrs. MacSorley was rushed to the ICU in a comalike state, having suffered some oxygen deprivation during her resuscitation. She remained on a respirator, unable to speak or to eat. The medical system was going all out to save her life.

At this writing, Mrs. MacSorley is still in the ICU, still on a respirator, and still unconscious. Not only is this case sad for the compounding of one tragedy on top of another, but for the lost voice of this patient. Going into the routine palliative surgery, Doris MacSorley had failed to be explicit about what she wished in the manner of terminal care. Her physicians all failed to anticipate the cardiac arrest. They then acted reflexively to save her life despite the fact that she was a terminal case. (There is, by the way, considerable discomfort among surgeons and anesthesiologists about not resuscitating a patient under these circumstances even if the patient had an active do not resuscitate order on the chart. Many feel that such an order is not binding in the operating room and therefore should be ignored or temporarily suspended so that there is no possibility of having to just stand by should an arrest occur.) In the absence of a clear plan for care, the juggernaut of high-tech curative medicine automatically slipped into gear. Instead of the patient's voice or an advance directive for care, the routine knee-jerk turning to high-tech medicine guided her treatment. In a sense, Mrs. MacSorley is trapped by the same system that seeks to treat her. She is totally dependent. Only her family can intervene to help her.

Suppose you were a family member or friend of Doris MacSorley's. How would you proceed? It is my hope that this chapter will give you some information as well as some food for reflection that will lead from this abyss.

Making decisions during an illness is not easy. The shock of sudden serious disease coupled with the demands of dealing with doctors, nurses, and relatives combine to produce a situation where events threaten to dictate the process of choice. When you enter the tangled, complex world of medical and ethical decision-making, it is like entering a deep forest. The growth is thick and lush, few maps exist, it is easy to get lost, and sometimes the dark and the unknown spaces can fill you with fear and foreboding.

These are the times to fall back on the powers of discernment and deliberation, taking time to reflect and to discuss, and perhaps develop a new kind of prudence and wisdom suitable for making sense of the new world of medicine.

This chapter will tell you about the terms of decision for many of the common problems encountered in critical-care medicine. Unfortunately, the answers are not here, but many of the questions are. And this is where to begin the search for a fitting response to the dark and perplexing choices that sometimes crowd into the souls of patients and their families.

Resuscitation

For the seriously ill patient, the question of cardiopulmonary resuscitation is one of the first value questions you will face in the ICU. Often the issue is avoided. The value at stake is the appropriateness of attempting to sustain life in the event of the sudden stopping of the heart and/or lungs. Research has shown that patients survive (that is, patients are well enough to leave the hospital) in only three to ten percent of all resuscitation attempts in general hospitals in the U.S. Ideally the physician should relate the medical facts and prognosis to you so that you may deliberate and decide the best course in light of medical information, life values, and personal preferences. Even when this ideal is not achieved before the ICU admission, the physician should ask you how he can best serve your values. The opportunity to ask may not come until the acute phase of an illness is over. But the physician's duty is to honor the autonomy of the patient. This means that the patient ultimately decides the extent and character of the medical treatment rendered.

But what if a patient is unable to communicate with his physician and has no written document expressing his wishes? Then the physician must turn to the family for assistance. Can the spouse supply a surrogate judgment of what the patient would want in these circumstances? Can other family members fill in a kind of character and value appraisal of the patient who cannot speak for himself? If the family declares that they know the mind of the patient (and who would better know?), then the question of pursuing or not pursuing a do not resuscitate (DNR) order would be settled. Spouses, sons, and daughters have a lifetime of intimate family history to fall back on for guidance. Living together through trials and exaltations, through good times and bad, is almost inevitably very revealing of a person's core values.

A do not resuscitate order can be written only by the patient's physician. The order would not allow the CPR techniques discussed in this book's appendix. Nor would it permit the so-called "slow codes" or "show codes" that are a sort of halfway measure, an unserious attempt to resuscitate done sometimes because of confused reasoning, ambivalence, or ethical doubts on the part of the caregivers. When a DNR order is properly written in a patient's chart, medical therapy is still maintained. Nothing about the care of the patient changes except in the event of an arrest of the heart or lungs. A DNR order should also be periodically reviewed by the patient, family, and care team. Some institutions have DNR orders that automatically expire at intervals, thus assuring timely review.

I can recall instances where the medical system itself has stood in the way of patients wishing to think seriously about a DNR request. Some professionals involved in the daily task of caring for critically ill patients thought that an informative brochure in the ICU family lounge would be an excellent way to get people thinking about not only the appropriateness of resuscitation, but other care issues such as advance directives and care of the hopelessly ill. Things went smoothly at first. Sample booklets from other institutions were gathered and evaluated. Finally a committee came up with a custom version of an informational pamphlet that was to be placed in all the critical-care lounges in the hospital. Readers of the brochure were invited to ask questions of the nurses and doctors in the respective units.

Everything went well until some of the surgeons who cared for patients in a cardiac unit objected to the content of the brochures. They thought it improper and psychologically harmful to raise the possibility of death to their patients. Some hospital administrators agreed with the surgeons. Seeing their institution as a palace of healing that competes with other institutions for market share, they saw it as most unseemly that their competitive position could be so undercut by mentioning the rude intruder—death. That is why they were against routinely asking all patients upon admission just what their values and attitudes were regarding ethics decisions should they become seriously ill while in the

CRITICAL CARE DECISIONMAKING

hospital. It was decided that families should be kept sheltered from any information with a negative connotation. The brochures never reached the patient lounges.

I can recall countless patients and families caught totally unaware in a medical situation that quickly went from bad to worse. Stunned by initial reports of bad news, the family is often paralyzed and unable to act. As I tell you this, I think of the Carlson family gathered around the hospital bed of their dying mother—a husband, two sons, and two daughters. They have flown in from the corners of the continent. Upon arrival, each hears the latest news and each responds with a measure of confusion and sorrow. Their mother's case drifts along. The several doctors involved are making all the decisions. No family member thinks to question them as each new tube or procedure desperately tries to stave off death.

Finally the visit of a life-long family friend galvanized the family to openly discuss their loved one's case and to think in terms of what might be best for the patient. What would *she* want done? Finding strength by relying on core family values and achieving group consensus, they were able to raise the question of a DNR order with the physicians. The doctors seemed relieved that finally this issue was in the open. They stated that they did not want to give up hope despite feeling for days that Mrs. Carlson had virtually no chance of recovering from her end-stage heart disease. Though Mrs. Carlson had suffered a cardiac arrest on two occasions during her hospital stay, both times massive interventions of drugs and defibrillation brought her back. To the relief of everyone, it was decided to attempt no more heroic resuscitation measures. The family, of course, felt very sad. But at the same time, they felt that the wife and mother they knew was no longer hopelessly mired in mindless, unlimited medical technology.

CHOOSING WISELY

A recent court case in Cincinnati demonstrates the perils of a DNR order on both the patient and the hospital. An elderly man was mistakenly revived with a defibrillator by a nurse who overlooked a standing DNR order. The man sued the hospital for the "wrongful" and miserable neurologically impaired life he had to live as a result of the resuscitation. The case underscores the growing trend of suits for overtreatment. This, of course, runs counter to physicians' traditional fear of being sued for not doing enough.

The crucial point to consider in do not resuscitate decisions is: Who decides and under what circumstances should a DNR order be entertained? Obviously the patient should have a primary role in this decision if he is able to understand the consequences and rationally contemplate this option with the advice of a physician and the family. If the patient does not have the appropriate decisional capacity, then surrogate decisionmakers should become involved. What is important is that patient and doctor know each other's mind regarding emergency care.

DNR orders are usually considered only in seriously ill or chronically debilitated or disabled patients who have no real hope of improving the quality of their experience of living. They are usually in obvious decline. Clearly they are on the glide path toward death. The decision to choose a DNR order is a means of avoiding fruitless and meaningless treatment. It reflects a wish to avoid prolonging dying. It is a recognition that death is not the ultimate enemy.

It is important to remember that there are fates worse than death. Being hung up between life and death, not quite alive and not quite dead, is a netherworld that you would best avoid if possible. Likewise, it is well to keep in mind that ultimately death cannot be cheated. Joseph Campbell, the renowned scholar of myth, reminded us about the meaning of the travail of suffering and death when he wrote: "The secret cause of all suffering is mortality itself, which is the prime condition of life. It cannot be denied if life is to be affirmed."

Withholding and Withdrawal of Treatment

Not everything that can be done should be done. After you confer with your care team, you will be in the best position to decide about what treatments are appropriate. One good way to make treatment decisions is to weigh the burdens versus the benefits of any proposed therapy. If the cancer chemotherapy will leave you nauseated, hairless, and weakened for its two-month duration, is it worth pursuing for a five percent chance of extending your life for five years? Suppose you have a failing heart. What would your life be like if you accepted heart valve surgery which would be risky, painful, and disabling throughout the long recovery period as opposed to the quality of your gradually deteriorating life without surgery? Again the balancing of burdens and benefits comes into play. Medical knowledge and statistics about outcomes might help your decision.

Some wise sense of the proportion of things also would be helpful. Is the contemplated treatment proportionate or disproportionate to the life values you hold? Do you believe that the therapy is not overkill or a technological attempt that ignores the human measure? Is the proposed treatment in congruence with the character and texture of the life you have so far lived?

Sickness uproots us from routine tasks and concerns. It dislodges us from the human community by upsetting and disrupting our habitual goals and expectations. The writer Flannery O'Connor, who suffered for years with lupus, said that being sick is like living in a foreign country—they do things differently there. The trick of making difficult decisions in the context of serious illness is in recognizing where the sick person has been, where he is now, and where he wants to go. This involves careful examination of and attention to the questions I have just raised about values and proportion and character. These are all elusive concepts that must be made concrete if we are to "rescue the person from the individual" in Thomas Merton's apt phrase.

In a sense this requires becoming a "knower of souls." You who are sick and you who care for the sick and you the person standing there looking at the side of your family member's bed, you must all work to achieve some kind of ripe and wise sense about the hidden center that is the core of the afflicted one. It is here that even the darkest and most befuddling questions of ethics can be addressed.

Quality of Life

The phrase "quality of life" seems to come up anytime ethical issues in health care are discussed. Withdrawing or withholding care frequently but not always carries the implication that such action may end in death. Since for most people, believers and unbelievers alike, life is not an absolute value but a value something less than the ultimate good, a very high value to be sure, it follows that there are some conditions where there are fates worse than death and where letting go is the preferred path to take.

The prudent person sees that death is part of life and that the values we live with endure beyond the flesh. So some sense of finitude is called for, the realization that life has a fitting beginning and end, and that our days on this earth are limited no

CRITICAL CARE DECISIONMAKING

matter what we think, do, or believe. The question we could ask ourselves that illustrates my point is: Would we really like to live in an endless present, repeating a certain way of living again and again, or do we acknowledge a certain longing to eventually move on from this world? To paraphrase the psalm: Teach us to number our days so that we may put on the heart of wisdom.

I remember when I was a medical student working in the emergency room. One evening I believed I encountered a family that had truly learned to number its days. The father was brought in and soon diagnosed with a heart attack. He was given the appropriate drugs and was hooked up to a heart monitor while awaiting his room in the cardiac-care unit. After the flurry of initial treatment the mother and her college-age daughter were allowed to come into the emergency room cubicle to see their loved one. I remember them physically holding each other, a mass of crying, quaking humanity there on the gurney. And then I remember feeling like an interloper just by being in the same place with them. They started to talk about the love that lived in their family. They felt impelled to exchange what struck me as last words with each other. They spoke as if the end were near. The possibility of death drew the family close around a warm center of loving concern. There was not a smidgen of denial or mawkishness or hysteria around the family. Their reaction to each other both attracted me and made me afraid. I hadn't given any thought that this fully conscious and alert man might die. And his family was reacting without the more typical numbed feelings and guarded optimism of most families I had seen. In retrospect, I see this family, whose name I do not remember, and the glimpse I had of them at this momentous time as blessed with a heart of wisdom, wise in their seeing of the numbered days. What I was also privy to was the wonderful and almost indefinable quality of being evident in how they related with one another. Something deeply and mysteriously human had happened in the little ER cubicle. It had been my privilege to see a small bit of the secret quality of life sneak out to the edges where I stood.

But how does one measure quality of life? This seems difficult enough in examining our own lives, much less coming to any conclusions about someone else's quality of life. But if we try to apply some common sense notion of what quality is in life, we may take at least one step in the direction of clarity.

Perhaps a quality life is a life where the self and others are esteemed and valued and where we live out and affirm what truths we can. Value is what gives our lives meaning; eating and conversation with friends, reading, lovemaking, thinking creatively, woodworking, gardening, weaving, snorkeling, bicycling, helping others—all these activities may make us feel more alive and connected to the life force. If they make us feel that way, perhaps other activities and experiences similarly give meaning to the lives of others. Despite the slippery nature of the phrase, quality of life becomes a very real consideration in the lives of seriously ill people who must make decisions about their care. If we choose not to use quality of life criteria, is there any grand principle or philosophy that will better serve us?

Though I know of many such principles and maxims and good books, I am somewhat of an existentialist on this problem in that I believe that the concrete particular experience of living produces the most persuasive argument of all. In the crisis of sickness, the voice of the patient is the experienced voice. And the quality of that experience, the quality of that life, is precisely the most wise, the most knowing, and the most appropriate person to decide those questions that are largely hidden from healthy others.

We are all in a certain sense the stories of our lives. As our own story unfolds, it reveals those values we have chosen for our lives. Perhaps one value of serious illness is that it peels away all the surface inessentials so that we can face our core selves.

Withdrawal from Treatment

A presidential commission studied the problem of foregoing life-sustaining treatment and issued a report in 1983. Though the members of the commission came from a wide variety of backgrounds and religious and philosophical persuasions, they were able to come to a consensus on how seriously ill patients should be treated. They stated forthrightly: Health care professionals serve patients best by maintaining a presumption in favor of sustaining life while recognizing that competent patients are entitled to choose to forego any treatments, including those that sustain life.

The American Medical Association has also published a statement on foregoing life-prolonging medical treatment. It says in part:

> The social commitment of the physician is to sustain life and relieve suffering. Where the performance of one duty conflicts with the other, the preferences of the patients should prevail. If the patient is incompetent to act in his own behalf and did not previously indicate his preferences, the family or other surrogate decisionmaker, in concert with the physician, must act in the best interest of the patient.
>
> For humane reasons, with informed consent, the physician may do what is medically necessary to alleviate severe

pain, or cease or omit treatment to permit a terminally ill patient to die when death is imminent.

So in dealing with doctors about your own or another's desire to exercise choice, remember that medicine has articulated some basic principles that support the patient's role in determining the limits of care. And it is also important to note that not every physician is aware of the extent of development of these principles. Many doctors still tend to see terminal-care decisionmaking as essentially a process that is legal rather than moral in character. Doctors may require a little nudging in the direction of sharing the burden of choice.

When you decide that further therapy is useless or insignificant and its cost is unduly harsh in terms of discomfort and suffering, you have reached a crossroads. If the decision is to back off from present care or to hold off additional care, the ethical result is the same. Sometimes caregivers and family members can agree not to start a particular treatment even if the treatment is medically advisable to sustain life. But the same doctors and family members often wince at the prospect of stopping therapy that is already under way to maintain the patient's life. Admittedly there is psychological stress in turning off a ventilator or disconnecting an IV. There is the appearance of actively doing something that will probably lead to the patient's death. Stopping treatment also can be seen as giving up, or stopping before a job is finished, or not doing everything possible to help. But on reexamination, it is the disease process itself and the patient's determination that enough is enough that are really the key elements that lead to the withdrawal of a burdensome treatment.

An additional problem in withdrawing a treatment is the chance that physicians will be reluctant to start an appropriate therapy because of their uncomfortableness in stopping it later

CRITICAL CARE DECISIONMAKING

down the road. This could lead to undertreatment. Appropriate use of high-tech medicine at those critical times in the disease- or injury-recovery process could be lifesaving. Everyone in critical-care medicine must sooner or later come to grips with the elusive distinction between prolonging life and prolonging dying.

I recall one situation where I was meeting with a newly formed hospital ethics committee at a medium-size hospital in Ohio. We were discussing the issue of withdrawing the ventilator support from a seventy-eight-year-old man who was suffering from ALS, or Lou Gehrig's disease, a condition that progressively weakens the muscles in the chest and diaphragm that move air in and out of the lungs. The gentleman, Horace Whitman, had been placed on the respirator three months earlier during a crisis in his battle to breathe. He indicated to his wife and to his doctors that he did not want to permanently live on an artificial breathing machine.

The question that arose for group discussion concerned how the physician and the ethics committee should respond to this case. Right away a physician in the group raised his hand and offered the opinion that to turn off the respirator would be equivalent to active euthanasia, in fact, he said, it would be like strangling the guy. I asked the doctor why he thought so. He related that the action of turning off a lifesaving device was tantamount to actively killing the patient.

The remainder of the evening's discussion at that hospital was a spirited consideration of the philosophical and practical problems of the case. Should the patient's wishes be respected? If Mr. Whitman were to die after turning off his respirator, would the more accurate cause of death be ALS or oxygen starvation? Does the intention of the caregivers make any moral difference in their actions or omissions? How does euthanasia, commonly understood as the direct, active, intentional ending of life under medical auspices, differ from the proposed withdrawal of the respirator in this case?

In Horace Whitman's dilemma, it took the active intervention of his very determined wife to eventually break through to the medical profession and honor his wishes to discontinue the respirator. Of course her intention was not to kill her husband. Rather, it was to respect his treatment choices and, together with her husband, bow before the powers of life and death that had dealt her husband a fatal hand.

Their decision acknowledges a higher power—that of Nature, a Creator—call it what you will. Their decision also recognizes that life is not an ultimate value but perhaps a part of a grander plan. The Whitmans refused to make an idol of biological existence. They saw the high moral and psychological costs of prolonging life beyond any reasonable biological boundary. At some point they decided that the wisest course was to acquiesce to death. Beyond a certain level of suffering and deprivation they did not view death as an enemy; further artificial means to prop up a failing life were interpreted as foolhardy and perhaps a little arrogant.

Futile Treatment

Finally, let's consider the healer's role and the notion of therapeutic futility. Under what circumstances should the practitioner back off and acknowledge that a cure for a particular disease is impossible?

If a proposed treatment seems futile, then starting or stopping it are ethically equivalent. The word *futile* is relatively imprecise—a slippery term having different meanings for different people.

CRITICAL CARE DECISIONMAKING

Physicians in one survey interpreted a futile therapy to be one that had anywhere from a zero to thirteen percent chance of success. What one person considers hopeless and without benefit, another will see as offering a remote hope. It is really a matter of prudent judgment as to whether a given therapy is being helpful. Futility perhaps is more easily recognized than defined.

One possible way to avoid initiating or continuing futile treatment is for the patient, family, and health-care team to discuss a time-limited trial of treatment. If the ventilator or tube feeding is to benefit the recovery of a patient from serious open heart surgery, or from the effects of chemotherapy in the case of a cancer, then time will tell how effective the therapy will ultimately be. It certainly is reasonable for the patient to give his medical intervention ample time to work. But it is also reasonable that there may come a time when it is apparent that a particular effort at healing and the reinstitution of health is simply not working. In this case, backing off seems appropriate.

The approach of the time-limited trial has many advantages. First, it breaks the impasse of deciding what to do. It also avoids the false alternatives of yes or no, all or nothing, this treatment or no treatment. Finally, it provides a built-in end point for a given therapy and escapes the pitfall of unrealistic treatment expectations stretching out into an indefinite future. The end of a trial could be a time for reconsideration or a recasting of the illness in terms of what has been learned during the trial of a new therapy.

The relationship between patient and caregivers and family is imbedded in a community context. What is considered futile is a cultural decision as well as an individual decision. Practitioners would do well to never assume that their patients see futile treatment through the eyes of medicine. Their vision is a close-up, intense personal experience of a life-threatening illness. Family will tend to see their afflicted member in the powerful terms of a relationship carried through time and now threatened by catastrophe. Any impulse on the part of the medical system to impose a solution in futile cases will lead to disaster. What will be destroyed is the trust in the relationship between the sick and the well, between the power of healers and the weakness of the ill. In the increasingly cost-accounting mentality of care, there will be even more temptation to ignore the patient and family's definition of futility and to impose a rational solution backed up by medical studies on outcomes of various diseases.

However, if the wider community arrives at an open and painful consensus about limiting care in certain situations, it is more probable that a patient and family will have expectations in care that fall somewhere in their comfort zone of what is acceptable to them. In Great Britain, for example, there is no societal expectation that dialysis will be started to treat the failing kidneys of a very elderly person. Therefore, no dilemmas arise in the care of Aunt Winifred, because patient, family, and practitioners, indeed the British culture, has arrived at a consensus of just what is appropriate.

The problem in tolerating another person's notion of futility is the very real possibility that they will make a "stupid" choice and thereby wastefully consume vast amounts of precious medical resources. If a patient is treated aggressively in the intensive care unit, the bed that he occupies will not be open for someone else needing total care. Since the number of beds and caregivers is not unlimited, you can see that choosing futile treatment may affect other people. Thus pressures to prevent futile therapy will grow amid the cultural chaos that now exists in American medicine. Since we have not yet arrived at a community consensus of how to face difficult care decisions, we end up with a series of individualistic treatment decisions and court cases that address the issue of futility.

Nutrition and Hydration

You will find no issue in bioethics more soul-wrenching than the problem of providing nutrition to the comatose or terminally ill patient. The availability of a technology that permits feeding patients who cannot eat has led to quandaries regarding proper treatment that have affected virtually every hospital and nursing home in the country. It is such a core issue in our culture that the Supreme Court in June 1990 rendered a key decision in the Cruzan case. This case involves a thirty-five-year-old woman from Missouri who was in a persistent vegetative state for over seven years following resuscitation after an automobile accident. Her parents petitioned the state of Missouri, and then eventually the Supreme Court of the United States, to follow their daughter's previously expressed wishes and allow her feeding tube to be disconnected. The case underscores the precarious balance, and indeed the ultimate mystery, between the forces of life and death, between deciding to live and deciding to die.

The Supreme Court decided that the state of Missouri has the right to protect its interest in human life by requiring that patients in the persistent vegetative state be kept alive. The court did grant that states have a right to stipulate their own requirements and exceptions to this general rule. The justices also said that a properly executed instrument expressing the wishes of the patient in regard to treatment would be valid. Implicitly the court rejected Nancy Cruzan's parents and other family members as surrogate decisionmakers. Instead, it established the very high standard of a written advance directive, even of a young person trapped in tragic circumstances. It appeared that as long as Nancy Cruzan resided in Missouri, she was as bound to its laws as she was to her feeding tube.

However, later in 1990 the attorney general of Missouri, having made his general point on behalf of the people, was moved to announce that the state would no longer oppose the Cruzan family's efforts if they petitioned the appropriate court to withdraw Nancy's tube. The family finally managed to accomplish this judicial goal. And so amid the harsh glare of the media and despite the interference of self-appointed "anti-euthanasia" groups, Nancy Cruzan's feeding tube was removed on December 14, 1990. She died twelve days later. But the moral implications and emotional turmoil of nourishing the critically ill certainly have not gone away.

Eating is fundamental to living. All of us were fed as infants and children. My mother nurtured me with chicken soup, ginger ale, and milk shakes when sickness interrupted my usual schooldays. I suppose at one time or another we have all been spoonfed and felt the care and concern of that person at the other end of the spoon. As we grow older we all tend to remember the good times we have had around the dinner table with our family celebrating a holiday or other special occasion. Later we might have memories of sharing a hamburger and french fries with an appealing person of the opposite sex. Still later we enjoyed candlelight dinners. And then there were wonderful feasts with friends —wine, wholesome food, memorable conversation. I could go on describing great meals at quaint restaurants or fresh trout over a campfire. My point is obvious. Food nourishes body and spirit. Feasting is an occasion to participate in the great human family. Food and the rituals of eating are rife with spiritual and psychological overtones. Whereas eating and sharing a meal are fundamental to our human natures, mere calories and the taking in of nutrition are restricted to a biological need.

All of this leads to the issue at hand. If someone—you, your father, your aunt—is afflicted by a stroke that has for all practical purposes extinguished that area of the brain that controls swallowing, and it is apparent after some months of rehabilitation that the ability to swallow will never be regained, then do you agree to have a feeding tube placed from which sustenance will be drawn?

Or suppose you are involved in an automobile accident and suffer a critical head injury that leaves you in that ambiguous halfway world we call the persistent vegetative state. Not being able to eat, do you want to be fed through a tube until death parts you from that tube?

Though on the face of it it seems extraordinary to feed someone through a tube, does that constitute extraordinary treatment? Or has technology, even relatively low-tech plastic tubes and a feeding mixture, totally abolished any notion of what is ordinary and extraordinary in medical therapy? What was extraordinary five or ten years ago is ordinary today; for example, pulverizing kidney stones with sound waves—unheard of a few years ago—is commonplace today. Though this therapy sounds like the stuff of science fiction, it is considered state-of-the-art care. So the terms ordinary/extraordinary do not seem to be of much help in elucidating this problem of feeding.

Likewise terms like simple/complex, usual/unusual, obligatory/optional, and invasive/noninvasive do not seem able to extricate us from the quagmire. As a patient, you might well decide to undertake a therapy that was either one or the other of these terms if you thought there was some chance of success and you were willing to bear the necessary burdens. So once again we come back to the concept of weighing benefits and burdens as a useful tool of deliberating about a proposed treatment.

In the case of tube feedings, I wonder if it also might be useful to think of this therapy as natural or artificial. We have already described the natural joys and conviviality of sharing a meal. In the case of tube feedings, this relational element is missing. Though tolerable in the short term in order to overcome a deficient or temporarily shut down gastrointestinal tract, a lifetime of tube feedings might well be unacceptable, as it is unnatural and artificial and unenjoyable. It also underscores that the reality is that such a patient has a fatal pathology—an inability to chew and swallow, and, in some cases, to digest food. In the same sense that a failed heart or failed kidneys may lead to optional treatment with an artificial heart or kidney, a failed GI system may lead to artificial feeding. Whatever the case, it is your option to decide whether and how long to accept such treatment.

If you opt not to accept artificial nutrition, how are you to squarely face the pain and suffering that this decision may cause. I think there are a number of steps that can be taken by talking to the doctors and nurses about these issues. Once a patient forgoes life-sustaining treatment, this does not mean that all care has been forsaken. In fact, from the health-care team's point of view, the emphasis has shifted from curing to caring. Problems that might arise in regard to pain control can be solved with appropriate drugs. The alleviation of suffering, that is, the psychological distress and displacement and alienation of illness, depends on the loving support of family, friends, and caregivers.

If oral intake is impossible, then the question is whether IV fluids should be administered. Without any fluid intake, dehydration would occur in a matter of days, though it is unclear if dehydration is particularly painful or thirst-inducing in the dying. Oftentimes hospice workers have observed that dying patients voluntarily decrease fluid intake. Comfort measures for the lips, the mouth, and the throat in the form of gels, ice chips, and sprays can alleviate the discomforts associated with no oral intake.

Some patients may prefer the infusion of an IV solution and feel better because of it. IVs can be given on a periodic basis through a heparin lock, which is nothing more than a short piece of tubing that stays in the arm and can be easily accessed periodically with the IV needle. Other patients find that keeping their body fluids up to a near-normal level increases the amount of respiratory secretions, which in turn increases discomfort in its own way.

Sometimes patients and families will disagree with their physician about withdrawing treatment. I recall one family who had been told by their physician that he would not participate in "starving" their grandfather and therefore would not discontinue his feeding tube. This was despite the patient's and family's clearly stated wishes after long and painful consideration. Further, the doctor stated, he would not open himself up to criminal or malpractice charges.

When I talked with the family, they were both devastated by this multiplication of suffering and very angry at the physician. I pointed out to them that the doctor had punched all the right buttons to blunt and immobilize their plans for caring for their grandfather. Invoking the word *starvation* immediately put the family on the defensive and made them feel slightly ghoulish. And then wrapping himself in the blanket of the law made the physician feel self-righteous. The family once again was left with the feeling that they were proposing something vaguely illegal and certainly not in the best interest of their grandfather.

I counseled the family to see the basic unfairness of the physician's attitude. It soon became clear to me and to the family members that this particular physician's analysis of their grandfather's case and his general discernment of the core issues of autonomy and prolonging dying were very wanting. I told them I also thought the doctor's reaction signaled his own discomfort, fear, and lack of facility in dealing with these very troubling issues.

My advice to this family was obvious—transfer the care of their grandfather to another physician, another hospital if necessary. Experience has taught me, however, that this simple solution is not always obvious amid the turmoil of terminal illness. Often patients and family are bound to their physician in a most unnatural way. Divorce seems unthinkable, even in the face of such a fundamental disagreement in care as I have described. And since the issue is care and the alleviation of pain and suffering, it is prudent to think hospice rather than hospital in terminal situations. So if the care is unsatisfactory, have a family meeting, openly discuss the dilemma, and do not fear dissolving a professional relationship and establishing a more sympathetic one.

The decision to withdraw or withhold a treatment calls us all to redefine and redescribe the core values of our lives. That we are more than a mechanically functioning collection of biological systems is obvious to all but the most ardent vitalists. Their argument is for the preservation of any life at any cost—a kind of idolatry of the body as an absolute value. Leon Kass, a doctor who teaches and writes about ethics, offers an antidote to this kind of rigid thinking: "The center of medicine has not changed: it is as true today as it was in the days of Hippocrates that the ill desire to be made whole; that wholeness means a certain well-working of the enlivened body and its unimpaired powers to sense, think, feel, desire, move, and maintain itself. . . ."*

Another physician, Conrad Rosenberg, captured what it feels

---

* Leon R. Kass, "Neither for Love nor Money: Why Doctors Must Not Kill," *The Public Interest*, 94(1989):39.

like to be caught like a cipher in the machine of technomedicine in his poem *How Do I Sign?**

> Water me no more
> with glucose and saline,
> I am pod not seed,
> I will not bloom.
> And puff me no more
> with oxygen.
> The monitor's beam
> may dance on the screen
> forever fed by
> your green tanks and bottles,
> your plastic tubes and pumps
> mimicking order, but
> I am chaos.
> The respirator reaches out,
> seizes my throat,
> chokes all speech.
> Mute, my thoughts show
> on no screen.
> How do I sign
> "Let me go"?

* *The New England Journal of Medicine,* May 10, 1990, v.322:1400.

States of (Un)consciousness

The intensive care unit typically treats persons who range widely in the state of their consciousness and the degree to which they can relate to the external world. Furthermore, the same patient may travel widely between different states of consciousness, even in a given day and night. Since awareness of the world, indeed wakefulness itself, is centered in a particular area of the brain, quite naturally insults that affect that area of the brain—trauma, drugs, toxins, infections—cause both familiar and unfamiliar, mild and profound changes in consciousness. We will review several of these altered states and see what application they might have in making informed ethical decisions.

Coma is the familiar term used in movies and books that brings to mind many a medical drama. Coma is a state of unconsciousness where a patient cannot be aroused even when painful stimuli are applied. In the coma condition the patient appears to be sleeping without interruption.

In the condition referred to as the persistent vegetative state (PVS), the patient is essentially unconscious, unarousable, and unaware of his surroundings, though painful stimuli may elicit a grimacing or a withdrawal response. Since the PVS person's lower brain performs well, breathing, heartbeat, digestion, and other vegetative functions go on indefinitely if food and fluids are supplied. However, voluntary actions such as swallowing and higher brain functions like thinking, learning, and remembering are lost.

Since higher cortical functions are absent in the PVS patient, the condition is often referred to as cognitive death. The PVS victim does go through sleep-wake cycles and can open eyelids, though the eyes do not focus or follow. Because the experience of pain involves the high centers of the brain, PVS patients can neither appreciate their plight nor experience pain at more than a reflexive level. In fact, it is difficult to conceive of a PVS victim as experiencing being at all. Since the higher brain is dead, no relating to or cherishing of other human beings is possible. It is naturally impossible to fully enter the consciousness of a PVS victim, yet to see them as beings without human brains, save the lower brain which automatically carries on bodily functioning, is not to deny that they are still a variety of human being.

To be diagnosed in the persistent vegetative state, a period of weeks to months of limited neurological functioning must have elapsed. In the United States today there are estimated to be from fifteen thousand to twenty-five thousand persons with this diagnosis.

The Carmen Mosher Case

The duties of care owed to a person in the persistent vegetative state are, of course, central in the Supreme Court's consideration in the Cruzan case. For all the notoriety of this case, it certainly is not unique. When I was associated with a large medical center, I came to meet a thirty-year-old woman who had recently delivered her third child. Carmen Mosher never was able to appreciate her lovely infant daughter, for soon after delivering, a large cerebral aneurysm, or ballooning artery, burst in her brain. She bled profusely inside the substance of her brain.

Despite the quick evaluation and intervention by a neurosurgeon, the brain hemorrhage devastated the person known as Carmen Mosher. As I watched her in her hospital bed, I saw the shell of a young woman, head shaved, eyes closed with twitching eyelids as if she were dreaming or struggling with an impossible idea. Her head would move from side to side on her pillow, back and forth, back and forth. Calling her name or touching her hand evoked no acknowledgment, no response. The portable radio on her bedside table played upbeat rock music for itself. Carmen Mosher was away from the world in which she had lived her previous thirty years. Her husband and children could no longer enter her consciousness. She did not respond to the world except to cringe occasionally and to open her eyes without seeing. After months of tests, attempts at rehabilitation, and the constant attention of her husband, Carmen Mosher was diagnosed as a person in the persistent vegetative state. Artificial feeding with a gastro tube had been instituted early in her illness when there was still hope for neurological recovery. The feedings that had once sustained hope now nourished a grim pessimism.

It was at this point that Vincent Mosher, her husband, began probing her doctors for some sort of signal that they saw what he saw. A former geography teacher and now an assistant junior high principal, he knew very early on the dimensions of the tragedy that had befallen his family. He was struck not only by the sheer awesomeness of the situation, but by the sensation of an intertwined fate with another couple they had read about in the newspaper on whom the exact same burden had fallen. Another sudden brain hemorrhage. Another woman left cut off from the world. Carmen and he had discussed this case which had occurred two years previously. And with a sureness of a young woman with practically her whole adult life in front of her, Carmen told Vincent that if the same thing ever happened to her, she would not want to be hooked up to tubes and imprisoned in such a life. No, she definitely would not want it.

Remembering this discussion with his wife, there followed a period of doubt, followed by a time of exasperation for Vincent

CRITICAL CARE DECISIONMAKING

Mosher. The doubt came to him in the dark days before he decided to approach Carmen's doctors with a plan to respect his wife's wishes and withdraw the feeding tube and allow her to die peacefully. The exasperation came after weeks of temporizing, talking, and reluctance on the part of the doctors. Were they struggling too, he wondered. Or was there something about being a surgeon that would not permit a defeat by death? Finally, after much conversation and soul-searching, after seeing lawyers and ethicists, after more confirmatory tests about brain function, the care team agreed to remove his wife's feeding tube according to her wishes. Carmen Mosher continued to receive hydration through an IV. She died three weeks later.

In a sense, the Mosher case was easy from an ethical point of view, given the clear expression of choice by the patient. But think of how much more difficult it would have been had she not spoken to her husband or had the hospital refused to honor her request.

Other potential problems with PVS patients have to do with the accuracy of making this diagnosis. The question of how truly persistent the condition is has come to light recently in at least two cases where the person judged by expert neurologists to be PVS has awakened. Persistent may in rare cases not be permanent. As if it were not already difficult enough to decide how to treat and for how long, the possibility exists that medicine's ability to diagnose PVS is fallible. The accomplishment of an ethical consensus on these questions has a limited tolerance for imperfection. Family and doctors are left suspended in the twilight zone of doubt, while the patient is left somewhere between life and death.

There are many ways to think about PVS patients. Two images come to mind. There is the image of the exile—a person banished from the world of human relations and ambitions, fated to live out life in a remote and strange place. There is also the image of the missing person, perhaps an amnesiac, lost in space and time, cut off as well from the fond and familiar. Both images have in common a cataclysmic disruption of the ordinary frame or pattern of living; when a person's place in the context of the human community is lost, the integrity of social relations disappears. The PVS being is not all here, not entirely with us. It is open to debate about which is the greater mystery—the part that is missing or the part that remains with us.

Still, I think there is some practical advice that might be helpful in the midst of such painful tragedy. If a family member or a friend is diagnosed to be in the persistent vegetative state, the time-limited trial of all-out therapy and rehabilitation may help to resolve dilemmas of care. Certainly six months of maximum treatment, perhaps a year in some cases, will give sufficient time for evidence of hope to arise. This would be time to see if any neurological function is regained. If despite an intense effort to reach into someone bound in the PVS is unsuccessful, a certain clarification will have occurred over this time that might serve to guide families in determining how to proceed.

Palliative Care

Once you have moved from the domain of disease, and fighting and searching for a cure, you arrive at the place where the essence of nursing and doctoring happen. This is the place where one human being cares for another—the fundamental transaction of the healing professions.

Palliation means to cloak or conceal the rough intensity of a disease. It means to relieve, to comfort, to bless those who are suffering. To do this well requires first of all the skill and sensitivity to recognize and to acknowledge the process of dying. After this is done, the considerable resources of medicine and nursing can be employed to soothe and relieve the dying person.

Pain can almost always be abolished with the use of potent drugs. The liberal use of narcotics, if possible, under the direct control of the dying patient herself, is extremely effective. The practice of patient-controlled analgesia, or PCA, is a very promising development in pain control. This system of IV pain relief allows the patient to self-administer a pain-relieving dose of medication. The system can be programmed with safeguards that would prevent inadvertent or intentional overdosing of drugs. Some studies have shown that when control of pain medication is turned over to the patient, it engenders psychological benefits, explicitly acknowledges the patient's self-determination, and often leads to a decreased total dose of the pain-relieving drug.

Though the dying patient does not have to worry about becoming addicted, some worry nonetheless. I once cared for a dying woman with lung cancer who refused to take narcotics with names she recognized like cocaine and morphine, because in her mind these were the substances used by dope fiends and street criminals and she didn't want her family and friends to associate her with those drugs. I remember the determination on Mrs. Carelli's face when she told me that she would prefer more physical pain if she could avoid the embarrassment of being a drug addict. The problem was resolved by giving her a potent narcotic that did not have a reputation on the street or in the news. This was acceptable to Mrs. Carelli and effective in making her final weeks physically comfortable as well as morally palatable.

Occasionally pain is so intense and unremitting that narcotic drugs have to be used in higher and higher doses. This has the effect of not only relieving pain, but sometimes it "snows" the patient into unconsciousness or into a waxing and waning semiconscious state. With very large doses of narcotics, the brain center that drives respiration is depressed. This means that a very delicate situation may develop when the doctor prescribes high-dose pain relievers that come perilously close to cutting off the dying patient's desire to breathe. Too little drug means pain. Too much means death. It is precisely here that the thin line between killing and letting die evaporates. For some ethicists, intention is morally crucial. Was the drug given to relieve pain or to kill by overdose? The answer to the question can establish a crucial moral distinction. The will to relieve pain is separate from the will to end a patient's life.

Surgery and X-ray therapy can also be used to provide comfort for the dying. A painful bowel obstruction or a growing tumor mass pressing on a nerve are examples of situations where these modalities might be extremely helpful.

Hospice

Finally, it is literally impossible to talk about palliative care without mentioning the hospice movement. The organizers of and volunteers of hospice are experts at providing comfort to the dying. Their services can make all the difference in the comfort and dignity of a person's final days. The aim of hospice is to support the entire family who suffer and grieve with their dying loved one.

The fundamental orientation of hospice is the belief that death is not the enemy. Death is rather seen as an inevitable place where all humans must travel to and through. "We give birth astride a grave," said Samuel Beckett, and this knowledge of our impending fate underlines the only certainty of our days on this earth. The knowledge of our own death raises fundamental spiritual and psychological and physical issues to which the hospice movement, through vast experience, is acutely sensitive. Physician and teacher Leon Kass eloquently writes about the place of death in modern medicine:*

> Even the most healthy human being must someday die, despite all efforts of the most competent physician. Such it is to be a mortal being, and such it is to have but extremely limited powers. Physicians need to accept these lessons no less than anyone else. If medicine takes aim at death prevention, rather than at health and the relief of suffering, if it regards every death as premature, as a failure of today's medicine, but avoidable by tomorrow's, then it is tacitly asserting that its true goal is bodily immortality. Once it is put that way, it should be clear that physicians must teach themselves and their patients to make their peace with finitude.

Brain Death and Death

Nowhere is there more confusion in the public mind than about the precise meaning of the term *brain death*. The human brain consists of two levels—higher and lower. The higher cortical centers of the brain are the areas involved in thinking, speech, and the coordination of complex muscular movements. The

---

* Leon R. Kass, "Practicing Prudently," in *Toward a More Natural Science*, The Free Press, New York, 1985, p. 205.

lower brain stem, or animal brain, controls spontaneous breathing and reflexes and digestion—in effect, the body's automatic pilot for carrying on basic life processes.

When both levels of the brain are rendered inoperative, be it from trauma, stroke, poison, or lack of oxygen, the term *brain death* is often applied. Every state but Georgia recognizes that brain death is a term equivalent to death, that is, even if a heart beats and respiration is maintained, either artificially or naturally, but it can be demonstrated that *both* the higher and the lower brain are irreversibly not functional, such a person, by the so-called Harvard brain-death criteria, is dead despite appearances to the contrary. The appearance of a rising and falling chest with respirations as well as a steady heartbeat and pulse belie the irreversible and permanent damage that has been done to the brain.

But the breathing and heartbeat run directly counter to the older and more familiar criteria of death, which is the permanent cessation of circulatory (heart) and respiratory (lung) functions. We are all very familiar and comfortable with this commonsense way of determining the end point of life. When death often occurred in people's homes, this is how it was decided that Aunt Cassie was dead there in her favorite chair in the sitting room. This convention was reinforced at the movies where the death of countless cowboys, Indians, and gangsters was signified by last gasps and absent heartbeats. If the person was not breathing and didn't have a heartbeat, that person was, by societal agreement, dead.

The whole-brain-death criteria established in 1968 are confusing to many because of the disturbing appearance of a loved one breathing and with a heartbeat who is nonetheless said to be dead. Technological intervention in the form of artificial support for respiration, nutrition, and kidney function, combined with potent drug stimulation of the heart, allows bodies without functioning brains to continue physiological survival for a time. This

CRITICAL CARE DECISIONMAKING

support may buy time so that solid organs—heart, liver, and kidneys—may be taken from the brain-dead corpse.

The phrase *brain-dead corpse* is an intentional redundancy that I have created to illustrate the intrinsic paradoxes technology has spawned. Such a corpse is distinguishable from another redundant entity, the "dead corpse"—i.e., one declared so by the more traditional heart-lung criteria—only because of the artificial life supports sometimes employed temporarily with the "brain dead." The "brain-dead corpse" may take on the appearance of being alive if the latest medical technology involving mechanical functioning of organs is applied. Sometimes in ICUs, nurses take care of brain-dead patients, which is to say that nurses, for a time at least, take care of dead persons as if they were alive.

Can you imagine what must run through the mind of a nurse caught in such a situation? Schooled in providing care and comfort to patients as well as regulating drugs and technical devices designed to support life, the nurse is asked to continue such care to a person/patient who in the morning is a critically ill ICU case and in the afternoon is an artificially maintained nonperson/cadaver. Mind you, nothing in the appearance of the occupant of the bed has changed. The chest rises and falls. The heart beats on. The IVs are running. Medications and nutritional support is still given.

It is easy to imagine some doubt creeping into the mind of the nurse. Is this being really dead? What has changed from morning to afternoon beyond the declarations of the doctors? The line between life and death becomes blurred. To survive as a caregiver, the nurse must truly *believe* in the Harvard whole-brain-death criteria. But the eyes argue against the mind. A surreal pretense must be maintained as the organ harvesters wait in the wings. The person is dead; the body lives on. One must sympathize with the nurse in this struggle at the edge of life.

It is important to distinguish the difference between the PVS patient and the patient who under the Harvard criteria is dead. PVS patients are able to maintain lower brain functions that control the basic physiologies of the body. Their hearts beat without the aid of powerful cardiac drugs, the vasopressors, and they breathe without the aid of a respirator. However, the higher cortical functions are absent—the rational centers and the centers which make possible both self-awareness and the experiencing of pain.

With whole-brain death the lower brain functions are absent in addition to the cerebral or high-brain functions. In order to determine whether a patient meets the whole-brain criteria of death, a rigorous neurological examination is necessary. Specialists in the nervous system, neurologists, generally conduct this kind of evaluation.

Their first thought is to rule out possible causes of unconsciousness that are reversible. Drug poisonings, metabolic disorders, hypothermia, shock, and cold-water drownings, especially in children, will all set off a cautionary response in the evaluation. Basically there has to be clinical evidence of deep coma over time, with a demonstration of no electrical activity in the brain or blood flow to the brain. In addition, reflexes normally controlled by the brain stem such as bright light constricting the pupils of the eye or gagging in response to stimulating the back of the throat are absent on testing. It is also important to check for spontaneous respirations, since this would be indicative of some lingering brain-stem function and thus is incompatible with the whole-brain criteria of death. Testing for the lack of respiratory drive is carefully carried out with the neurologist, paying close attention to the mixture of gases being breathed through the respirator and the amount of time the patient is taken off the ventilator in order to assess spontaneous respiration.

Results of this kind of testing are not always predictable. When Karen Quinlan was removed from her respirator, the expectation, following the years of family pain and judicial review, was that she would immediately succumb. She lived for more than nine years off the respirator. (She therefore was in a persistent vegetative state and was not brain dead at the time she was taken off the ventilator.)

There is not universal agreement in our society about the Harvard whole-brain criteria of death. Everyone seems to agree that when a person's heart and lungs irreversibly cease working for more than three minutes or so, that person is dead. However, Orthodox Jews and other religious groups have challenged the adequacy of whole-brain death as a definition of death. Others have questioned the motives of the medical establishment's imposition of a new definition of death. These critics suggest that these new criteria are expedients created to make possible the donation of organs for transplantation. Solid organs quickly lose their ability to work if they are cut off from their blood supply for too long. In order to be useful for transplantation, the donor organs in the cadaver must be maintained on artificial life supports to assure viability at the time of "harvesting" for the recipient of the transplant. Without whole-brain-death criteria, very few organs would be available for transplantation.

It might be helpful to think of death as a process that unfolds on a continuum that starts with a healthy person who ages, sickens, weakens, becomes unconscious, and eventually stops physiological functioning. Society decides at what point in this dynamic process of deterioration death should be declared. It does this on the basis of the pragmatic and psychological needs of the human family. Death is neither defined as the point when someone becomes unconscious or the point at which the flesh begins to rot. Rather, it is said to occur by cultural consensus at some point, or, in our present situation, two possible points, where our own societal values have concluded that life is at its end.

I know this is all very complicated, and obviously the stakes in deciding what is living and what is dead are very high. But I think one of the major tasks of the patient and family in the ICU is to get to know death better—not only in regard to the technical details I've been talking about, but in all the religious, philosophical, and psychological richness possible for an individual to absorb. Reflecting on these matters, talking forthrightly with others, perhaps doing some reading on the subject—all this contributes to meeting the prospect of death with open eyes. The worst possible course is to ignore or deny the subject of death.

I have seen numerous families caught up in denying the obvious. Often the doctor is an accomplice in maintaining an air of unreality about a death that is coming. I recall one family in particular who would always ask me after visiting Mr. Josephson, "Don't you think he looks better?" The patient was slowly dying from liver cancer and to me looked to be deteriorating at a rapid rate. His yellow cast and hollow cheeks strongly suggested a dreadful outcome. But the family persisted in seeing their relative in an entirely different way. The manner in which they couched their questions was really a way of fending off discussion of their loved one's impending death. They obviously were not ready to talk about death or any other terminal-care-treatment issue. It was a delicate situation. No one wanted to bluntly break through to the family and destroy a sustaining illusion about themselves or the patient. At the end, some days later, they pretended that his death was a surprise.

The Euthanasia Debate

In the intensive care unit you cannot help but notice that suffering, despair, and defeat are common visitors. In the midst of pain, hope is sometimes lost. The body lingers. It will not heal. It will not die. At times like these, thoughts of the end of life may come to dominate the mind of the gravely ill person. One may ask why all this pain and suffering? Why me? The patient may look to the nurse and the physician for relief from their terminal trial. They may ask for assistance in ending their own lives.

The euthanasia debate has appeared and reappeared in our country through the years. Derek Humphry's recent best-selling book of death-dealing recipes has captured the attention of a very large number of readers. The book and the discussion it has sparked are the latest surfacing of the euthanasia question. The last decade has also seen intense interest in the so-called right to die and in the Dutch experiment with active euthanasia. In Holland in recent years physicians have been dispatching terminally ill patients, perhaps five thousand per year, usually by administering a drug overdose. The practice is intended only for those who voluntarily agree to die. Although the killing is technically illegal, prosecutors have chosen not to pursue cases that conform to medical criteria established by the profession and that are openly brought to the attention of authorities by proper notification on the death certificate.

Kurt Vonnegut wrote of "ethical suicide parlors" in one of his futuristic fantasy stories of the early 1970s. These places of his imagination were where the old and feeble were expected to go and die peacefully in a decorous atmosphere with appropriate refreshments and music. Less than twenty years later, Vonnegut's playful musings seem more like a prophecy.

In the United States, direct, active euthanasia is illegal in all jurisdictions. The extent of the underground practice of euthanasia is unknown. Persistent reports that some physicians participate in the killing of patients who request to die are seemingly regular items in the press. Still, very few physicians are open about their own beliefs or practices regarding the taking of life.

By euthanasia I mean the active taking of a life with full intent to end a life by a quick and painless means, usually an overdose of drugs that overwhelms the brain and delivers a patient to rapid unconsciousness and thence to cessation of bodily functions. The motivation is usually the alleviation of serious pain by bestowing "mercy." This practice should be distinguished from withdrawing or withholding life-sustaining treatment. This kind of decision does not intend the death of the patient, nor does it provide the means of death. It is rather the humble acceding to powers outside of medicine and to the hope that dying should not be prolonged with fruitless therapy.

Proponents of euthanasia make their argument on two principal grounds. First, on the basis of autonomy—the individual's right of self-determination in matters relating to his or her own body. In a sense, the argument runs, our bodies belong exclusively to ourselves. Therefore, no familial, social, or religious claims can abridge this right. We are free to decide the time of our own death in the context of a grave illness or debility. The kind of control over dying inherent in this argument is in direct opposition, and perhaps a reaction against, the power that doctors and hospitals currently exercise over the death process. Seen as part of a wider grass-roots consumer movement in this country, the right to die movement similarly uses politics, the media, and the courts to try to achieve its ends.

The second basic argument for euthanasia states that there are certain situations where because of terrible suffering, intractable pain, or total loss of human dignity, life is not worth living. The lack of quality in a life so diminished leads a person to opt for death. A planned death thereby eliminates suffering, avoids the embarrassment and vulnerability of illness, and affirms autonomy.

Opponents of euthanasia argue that human life is a sacred gift and trust, that our lives really are voyages of stewardship, and that to respect the sanctity of life one must not intend to end one's own life or the life of another. To do so would violate a fundamental human value and cheapen the life that God or nature has given us. To do so would be insulting to the giver and demeaning for the recipient of the gift of life. In short, the argument goes, our lives are *not* entirely our own.

The other principal argument against euthanasia involves the roles inherent in the healing professions. To profess nursing or medicine is to offer assistance and care to the needy and vulnerable sick. It is to take on professional values and to commit oneself to making people whole, to relieving suffering, and, ultimately, to bowing to powers beyond the scope of the healing arts. Immense damage to the relationship of trust between doctor and patient would be done if the doctor who healed was also the doctor who in some circumstances killed. So goes the argument that even if our society developed a consensus that euthanasia was a good policy, doctors and nurses could not afford to confound their traditional responsibilities.

Other critics of euthanasia point out that once voluntary euthanasia is started, it is a very slippery slope to involuntary euthanasia of the undesirable, the troublesome, and the incapacitated. Often the history of Nazi euthanasia in Germany in the 1930s is cited as evidence that once the feeble-minded and deformed are euthanized for some laudable improvement of the human race, the concept of a "life unworthy of life" can lead to the devastating consequences of mass extermination. The Nazi specter of eliminating the retarded, the congenitally disabled, and the mentally ill in the late 1930s, before the Holocaust was implemented against the Jews, is the millstone argument around the neck of euthanasia advocates. History is hard to fight, especially when it has occurred within the lifetime of so many people who are now nearing the end of their natural lifespans.

But you would think for the average person, Dachau and

Auschwitz are somewhat remote as they face the anguish of severe illness. In a possibly terminal situation, it is imperative that the care team be alert and responsive to issues of suffering and pain, and dying and death. It seems obvious that far too few physicians are adept at attending the dying and using drugs that will promptly and effectively relieve pain. Inadequate control of this type of pain, writes one authority, "exacerbates the suffering component and demoralizes the family and caregivers who feel they have failed in treating the patient's pain at a time when adequate treatment may have mattered most."* The best estimate is that fully two-thirds of the cancer patients in the United States in the advanced stages of their disease suffer significant pain—pain that is often unrelieved.

The euthanasia movement is partially fueled by the desire of many patients to reassert some control over their own lives as they are lived in hospitals. In a sense, the movement is a revolt against impersonal, technological medicine. Proponents of euthanasia also take advantage of the very natural and understandable fear of pain that we all have. If one loses the power to abolish or at least control pain, then one might entertain the idea that the solution is in eliminating the life that so pains.

Assisted Suicide

When a health-care professional engages in deliberate actions that would tend to enable, instruct, or encourage a patient to end his own life, the caregiver in effect is assisting in the ending of

---

* Foley KM, Arbit E. "Management of cancer pain," in DeVita DT, Hellman S, Rosenberg SA, eds. *Cancer: Principles and Practice of Oncology*, J. B. Lippincott, Philadelphia, 1989, p. 2064.

life. The physician or nurse assister of suicide is one step removed from the active taking of life. Assisted suicide is not quite active euthanasia. In this kind of scenario, the patient will typically ask the physician or other careperson to supply the means by which he can end his own life. If the physician supplies, for example, a lethal dose of drugs to a patient in the terminal stages of AIDS and provides instructions on how to most effectively use them, the physician violates the traditional view of the healing professions which view talk of suicide, or a suicide attempt, as meriting therapeutic intervention. Such intervention would be aimed at caring for the patient and at getting at the root causes of a life felt not worth preserving. The traditional view most assuredly would not look at a patient's request to die as an opportunity for a nurse or physician to validate a kind of personal autonomy that knows no bounds—an autonomy that has run amok.

The infamous Dr. Jack Kevorkian, a Michigan pathologist, demonstrated in 1990 just how ghoulish the business of physician-assisted suicide can become. Kevorkian rigged up an IV with deadly drugs and then turned the controls over to an Oregon woman who was in the early stages of Alzheimer's disease. Following his instructions, the woman took her own life in the back of the good doctor's old Volkswagen van. There is no record or claim that Kevorkian offered any succor, support, care, or comfort to this very distressed woman. Rather, he seemed very intent on capturing the spotlight with his "suicide machine." He seems to have taken advantage of a very vulnerable woman in order to further his own campaign against what he sees as the shortcomings of the medical establishment's attitude toward death.

Kevorkian's encore caper in the fall of 1991 resulted in the death of two middle-aged women—one afflicted with multiple sclerosis, the other suffering from chronic pelvic pain secondary to a vague and not totally defined disease process. Neither woman was terminally ill. Neither woman was offered any meaningful hope, counsel, or referral for her problems. No disinterested third party or judicial authority or medical board oversaw or reviewed the process of death. Instead, Dr. Kevorkian boldly proceeded. He provided the means for their demise, and using the latest consumer technology, made a video of the women's final moments.

Dr. Kevorkian's actions occurred during the time the voters in the state of Washington were considering Proposition 119, the so-called "aid-in-dying" initiative. The proposal would have made it legal for physicians to give a deadly medicine to patients who requested it and who were terminally ill. The Washington proposal defined terminally ill to include those persons expected to die within six months. The second Kevorkian case hit the media just weeks before the vote in Washington was cast. This timing, in retrospect, was extremely important in influencing voters. Proposition 119 went down to defeat in a close vote. It seemed to have much initial appeal, but as discussion and debate went on, the public appeared to find more and more reasons to oppose this very radical departure from the prohibition against private killing. It is probable that Jack Kevorkian put a human face on the fears many voters had of giving the power to kill to an unstable or overzealous renegade doctor. In a curious irony, Dr. Kevorkian helped to defeat what he wanted most.

But the notion of assisted suicide can be less clear in certain cases. Suppose, for example, that a respirator-dependent homebound quadriplegic requests help in establishing the means of turning off his respirator by having a special switch installed that he could operate with his tongue. He wishes the switch not because he is entertaining thoughts of suicide, but because he wants to recapture some power over his life, a power all non-handicapped people take for granted. If the patient wishes to

CRITICAL CARE DECISIONMAKING

withdraw from ventilator treatment, he then would have the means to accomplish his end. Suppose that sometime after the switch is installed, the patient turns morose and declares that he no longer wants to live. He says he is sick of the respirator. Before his mood change can be adequately addressed, he switches off his respirator and dies. Did the health-care team assist in his suicide? Is the issue suicide, or is it a case involving withdrawal of treatment?

The year 1991 also saw the exposition of the case of Dr. Timothy Quill in Rochester, New York. Dr. Quill assisted a longtime patient of his who was in the final stages of cancer to end her life. He did this by providing the drug and the knowledge of how to use the medication to end life. He did so reluctantly and with great sorrow, and only after giving his best counsel and care to his patient. He tried to talk her out of it, but ultimately agreed with his patient, who needed control over her pain.

The case has two very interesting aspects. First, Dr. Quill wrote about the case and was published in one of the country's most prestigious medical journals, *The New England Journal of Medicine*. He wanted to be very aboveboard in what he was doing and the journal, too, wanted the discussion of the patient's and the physician's plight to become a public and professional policy question. Secondly, the issues of terminal illness, pain relief, and the notion of what kind of ultimate control we have about the manner of our passing were all vividly posed in the case of Dr. Quill. Here was a sensitive physician, not a fanatic or a publicity seeker, who described a poignant case where his decision to grant his patient "control" seemed a reasonable action. The question of why control seemed the dominant theme that Dr. Quill wished to serve rather than counseling humble acceptance or release is perhaps a larger question for our times. Where does this wish come from, to control even death?

Later in 1991 the public prosecutor declined to bring any charges against Dr. Quill. With regret, with sadness, and with reluctance, Dr. Quill aided his patient's dying. The forthrightness of his action and his unblinking determination to face and not flee from the issue are truly remarkable. But Dr. Quill has also blurred the traditional role of healer.

There are wider questions. Can you imagine your own physician actively participating in ending a patient's life? Would you feel comfortable putting your trust (indeed, trusting your life) in a doctor who would be willing to switch roles from healing to killing? Should your physician consider the taking of life as another "therapeutic option"? Similarly, would you be comfortable with a physician who might play an active role in medical executions in prisons? Your answer, of course, does not depend on whether you support capital punishment or not. The question is whether doctors should be willing to put their knowledge of anatomy and physiology and pharmacology in the service of death. Or would such action cross a crucial moral line? The twentieth century has seen many reports of physicians reduced to torturers, executioners, agents of the state, and now, dispatchers of the hopelessly ill.

What kind of social control can counter the immense power of doctors to decide who to heal and who to kill? Proponents of euthanasia and physician-assisted suicide offer few safeguards and no concrete mechanisms to oversee the carrying out of what are obviously very serious actions. Likewise, euthanasia apologists have very little to say about the inevitable mistakes in judgment that physicians will make about just who is truly terminally ill and about who is suffering intractable pain. Inevitably, a few unwilling or perhaps neutrally disposed individuals who happen to be poor and weak and sick and demented will be swept away by the kindly tide of benign death. And surely their dispatchers who mean well and who hope to stem the onslaught of suffering

CRITICAL CARE DECISIONMAKING

will themselves become brutalized in a process that blurs the line between standing and acting on behalf of life and acting with the arrogance of a god.

Death becomes a temptation, an easy solution in the face of complex pain and suffering. It is just one more technical fix to a profound human problem. It will not work because life more resembles art than it does technology. And healing involves more than the measurers can ever measure. Euthanasia and physician-assisted suicide are a flight from the demands of caring. If patients do not believe that the medical profession can provide adequate relief from pain and support through a grueling illness, then they, too, will be tempted toward the fast and easy exit from life. It is time for doctors to reassert their ancient and venerable goal of committing themselves to the alleviation of suffering, especially in cases where cure is no longer possible.

Physicians should also be clear about where the ultimate power of life and death resides—certainly not within the fallible limits of a human profession. Therefore, any attempt by a patient to hand over to the physician the power over life should be kindly and steadfastly refused. To request euthanasia or to ask a physician for help in self-destruction is to inappropriately give a power to another which is not yours to give, and not the doctor's role to receive. Turning our life over to another would be similar to a person agreeing to be another's slave. This kind of control over the life of another is repugnant. The damage done to both slave and master is mutually reinforcing—both parties are morally diminished. Life in its creation and at its core is too mysterious for any rational plan of destruction at its end to encompass. Remember that a medicine that is oriented toward biological existence alone knows little about the meaning involved in the full flowering of life in all its richness, surprise, and diversity. This is a higher realm altogether.

Twisting and distorting the ends of the profession of medicine is also extremely dangerous. Despite its shortcomings and failings, it is unrealistic to expect that medicine can retain its integrity by turning to the killing role when the healing role is unsuccessful. But the continuing debate on this topic underscores the notion that the ethical crunches in medicine tend to occur at the edges of life.

I hope this discussion helps you to realize the very knotty possibilities that can occur when autonomy and sanctity of life come into conflict. You can see that the wisdom of a Solomon may be required. And sometimes there is no universally acceptable answer, no way to serve the good that does not raise fears and doubts.

What is called for is what Aristotle called the virtue of *phronesis*. This is the capacity to rationally deliberate about a moral matter, to consider, to mull over the concrete circumstances of a case, and to arrive at a moral decision. Phronesis is practical wisdom. It is also discernment—the capacity to draw out and recognize the essential elements of an ethical problem.

Phronesis is a virtue developed through experience and conscious attention. Virtue-based ethics implicitly argues that as a person is, so shall he act. It has a vigorous confidence that the virtuous moral actor will act rightly. And it sees that reflective contemplation leads to a more fully realized rational person.

Experimental Therapies

Often the high-tech, sophisticated care we have been discussing is delivered in the university or other research-oriented medical centers. Often the very doctors who direct and teach teams of residents and provide bedside care are involved in research projects themselves. As part of their duties, they may be studying a drug or a combination of drugs that is not yet on the market. As professors of medicine, they are attempting to extend the range and the depth of medicine's understanding of a disease process or a drug effect.

Due to the abuses of the past in this country and the lingering ghost of Nazi experiments on human subjects, strong safeguards, including review boards, now watch over any medical trial involving humans. If you are to become a part of an experimental protocol, you must be duly informed and give your explicit consent.

The extent of human experimentation on unwitting subjects in the United States following World War II is still largely unrecognized. It was the publication of Dr. Henry Beecher's classic article, "Ethics and Clinical Research," in 1966, that not only gave birth to the movement in biomedical ethics, but was the first warning that human experimentation was not confined to a few criminal Nazi doctors.

Beecher documented and described twenty-two cases where dangerous and sometimes deadly experiments were performed on patients without their consent. A few examples to illustrate the abuses: Live cancer cells were injected into human subjects to study immunity to cancer; a small patch of malignant melanoma (an aggressive skin cancer) was transplanted to a young woman, leading 451 days later to her death from metastatic melanoma; high concentrations of nitrogen-containing substances were introduced into alcoholics suffering from cirrhosis, leading to clouding of their consciousness and tremors; among a group of military "volunteer" subjects with strep infection, definitive therapy with penicillin was withheld from some (they were given placebos) in order to study serious cardiac and kidney complications of untreated strep infections.

Twenty-five years of increasing consciousness about this problem has led to considerable reforms, but there are still at least two possible problems that individual patients must face in this regard. First, is it fair, if you are seriously ill, to expect you to consider the question of whether to participate in an experimental protocol given the extraordinary stress that you may already be under? Weighing burdens and benefits, considering alternatives, and pondering yet another complexity may be asking too much of some patients.

The second direct consideration is the question of whether there is a chance of any benefit by participating in an experimental trial. Often there is none. A patient might be asked to deviate from a treatment plan with established drugs that are known to work for, say, abolishing erratic cardiac rhythms, in favor of an experimental drug that may one day prove to be a better drug. However, the precise clinical effects, including possible toxicity, are unknown. In this case, the patient may or may not benefit from participation. In other situations patients will definitely not derive any benefit from an experimental protocol because they are involved at an early stage in a long series of experiments that will not produce clinical benefits for anyone for some years. Their only satisfaction might be the hope of advancing medical science one small step.

An ICU Strategy for Patients and Families

What you feared has finally happened. Your husband has suffered a massive heart attack and has been rushed to the hospital for emergency care. You think of the times you have exorted him to quit smoking and get more exercise. But it's too late for that

CRITICAL CARE DECISIONMAKING

now, and the fact that you may be right about what he should have done in the last ten years is of little comfort.

Things are now touch and go. Your husband has been admitted to the cardiac-care unit—a specialized intensive care unit for heart problems. The maelstrom of events and emotions clouds your thinking. What do you do? Where do you turn? You speak to your husband's cardiologist, a man you've never heard of or met before. He tells you that a sizable portion of your husband's heart muscle might have been destroyed by the heart attack. Time, he says, will eventually tell the true extent of the damage. He tells you that your husband is having difficulty breathing and may have to be intubated. He explains what this means. Meanwhile, your daughter has arrived from ninety miles away with her husband. You hug. You commiserate. The initial shock slowly dissipates and a heavy and dark realization moves in. Your husband is critically ill. He may die.

The situation I have described is everyone's nightmare. One could not think of worse circumstances under which to make crucial decisions. But the pressure of events will inevitably push the caregivers and the family into deciding very serious matters. What is the best plan for dealing with this situation? Obviously there are no easy answers. Books have been written about the intricacies of care and medical decisionmaking. What I would like to do is to suggest a general course and draw up a capsulized plan for facing the formidable concerns of making complex decisions under stress.

The first thing to do is to establish close contact with the afflicted loved one. Does your husband know the medical facts of his condition? Is it even possible at the early stages of treatment to approach him about the question of medical and ethical decisions? Is he too groggy, too drugged, too uncomfortable to entertain questions on the nature and extent of his future care? Perhaps it is best to back off at first and give him some time to regain strength. But this course is loaded with potential pitfalls. Suppose an important decision must be made before your husband is able to fully participate in care decisions. If he is not able to give consent and provide some guidance for his care, then just who does decide? You? The medical team? The entire family? Perhaps a collaboration of caregivers and family will serve the sick person best by seeking to give the kind of care your spouse would want were he able to speak for himself.

Has your husband previously expressed his desires about hospital care, either informally or through an advance directive? If so, this would be of great help in deciding the limits and scope of care. But if there is no previous statement to guide family and caregivers, is it possible to get to know the mind of this man while he is in the cardiac-care unit? Sometimes yes, sometimes no. There are times when a clouded state of consciousness will make such an inquiry impossible. Sometimes families are extremely reluctant to raise the issue with the seriously ill relative who is fully conscious and capable of discussing such issues. To avoid the issue is a mistake. Family members should seek to understand the mind and heart of their loved one so that they are clear about his goals and wishes regarding care. They should be prepared to back up his decisions when necessary. Though it may be difficult, never back away from an open discussion of the treatment issues. This means that the afflicted person must, before all others, be engaged in the process of decisionmaking about his care insofar as he is able to connect with the welter of events and concerns that swirl around his intensive care bed.

In order to make informed decisions about care, the latest and most relevant medical information must be at the disposal of the patient and family. This means staying in close touch with the nurses and doctors who are in and out of the cardiac-care cubicle.

CRITICAL CARE DECISIONMAKING

Ask questions. Seek specific information regarding prognosis, anticipated procedures, resuscitation orders, and duration of particular treatments such as respirators or dialysis. Ask what every tube is for. Stay close to the unfolding picture of your husband's illness. Know that the situation may change hour by hour, day by day. Ask to be informed about possible complications. Demand to be in on every major change in care *before* it is implemented (with the obvious exception of emergencies). Ask if surgery is contemplated. If doctors or nurses give vague answers to your questions, demand clarification. Be courteous, but do not hesitate to be persistent. Pester if you must. Your goal is to develop as complete a picture as you can glean about the medical condition of your loved one. This kind of information is crucial in order to be able to make informed decisions down the road. Your goal is also to be present in the collaborative care of your husband, to be seen as someone who speaks for your husband, representing him during informal conferences with doctors and nurses, participating in every crucial decision. This requires energy, alertness, and steadfastness at a time when you will be physically and emotionally drained yourself. The strain will cause you and your family to suffer with your husband. Part of you will want to scream and flee. At times you will think your task is impossible. You must know that to stand for and with your husband in his time of great need is the best way to help him.

You attempt to assure that what is done in the way of care is what your husband would want done. You stay in close touch with the medical and nursing care team. You seek their advice and knowledge; you are open to the wisdom of their experience in these matters. What more can you do as the days drag on? To fill the hours of waiting at the bedside or in the patient lounge, those who have a mind to can set about learning more on their own about a particular medical therapy, or about a troubling ethical problem that you see arising on the horizon. Tap into friends, confidants, and counselors; delve into books and helpful articles in the hospital library that may illuminate some aspect of your husband's case. All of this can be seen as useful work and as part of your husband's overall care plan.

Your efforts are meaningful and you will derive satisfaction knowing the decisions you and your husband and his caregivers make about critical treatment issues are based on substance and due consideration rather than on ignorance or pure emotionalism. Realize that though you cannot ultimately control your husband's fate or cardiac physiology, you can develop the requisite insight and understanding to see the terrible proportion of human vulnerability in the face of serious illness. And this is to see the human measure in life-and-death decisions and to know that doing your human best is all you really can do.

CHAPTER 4

Planning for Illness

"Sickness often creates a space to live in, freeing the mind from the habitual if only for a day or two. Ordinary stresses disappear and when one returns to usual routines everything seems a bit more clear though sadly the clarity quickly passes."
—Jim Harrison
Farmer

"The flesh is the spirit thickened."
—Richard Selzer

Alice and Bartholomew Swanson would always visit my office together. They were the quintessentially happy retired couple. Both had chronic medical problems—Alice with osteoarthritis, Bart with high blood pressure. But both Alice and Bart did not let their problems interfere with their enjoyment of life. They enjoyed each other. They enjoyed the time to pursue the things that gave meaning and satisfaction to their lives.

Alice was an omnivorous reader. Despite some vision problems, she read all the time and would delight in bringing in her latest book discovery or an article from *The New Yorker* for me to enjoy. Bart was dogged in his pursuit of trout. For him they were an occasion of joy. Every trip to his favorite northern Michigan stream was in his mind simply an acceptance of an invitation to spend some golden hours with the clear, gravelly waters, with the sweet smell of balsam, and with the brook trout that would grace his time in the stream. Like his favorite writer, Norman Maclean, for Bart "there was no clear line between religion and fly fishing."

Bart did not miss his past life as a police chief in a medium-size city. Alice, on the other hand, did miss the daily contact with her music students. They sensed that their lives were moving through time with what seemed like dramatically increasing speed. Like a stone dropped from a high cliff, the velocity of their remaining days seemed to be too rapidly heading toward its destination. They told me the feelings they were having with just a tinge of fear and regret. They were simply having too much fun to think too much about "the end."

In fact, the Swansons prided themselves on how well they had planned their lives. They had carefully planned the winterizing of their summer cottage so they could use it as a year-round home. They had carefully planned for the financial aspects of pensions, social security, and retirement funds. Together they had long-ago visited a lawyer and honed a will. Alice even made up a reading list for retirement that included every classic she had missed as well as all the modern books she had been meaning to read.

One day the Swansons came to my office with only one thing on their agenda. Bart and Alice told me of a friend who had suffered a devastating stroke and was in the hospital "all wired up and be-tubed." The family seemed paralyzed about making any decision about the patient's care. They did not know exactly what their friend wanted, but they knew what they would want. Both Alice and Bart had read about living wills. Their relative good health had made it easy to postpone any definite action to create such a document for themselves. Seeing their friend's situation dissolved any reluctance to go forward with some sort of instrument that would guide treatment in the event that they were unable to make decisions for themselves. There was no doubt that the Swansons could and would speak for themselves to guide their own medical care. As with everything else in their lives, they tried to anticipate problems.

Despite the wide publicity about living wills, the best estimates are that only ten to fifteen percent of Americans have actually taken the initiative to make an advance directive statement. True, there is widespread confusion about the content, the legalities, and the practical problems of going about constructing a living will. But that probably is not the whole story of why people seem somewhat reluctant about them.

Perhaps we should also consider the heavy philosophical, psychological, and spiritual aspects that you would face in making a living will. To even think about a living will, you must acknowledge that death is a certainty and that life has limits. In the midst of the joy and distraction of living in full stride, talk of dying, demise, and death is easily dismissed. Sitting down with a spouse or a physician or an attorney and speaking of these matters requires inviting a third party into your life as well—a rude and harrowing guest who never takes no for an answer. Naturally our inclination is to keep such visitors at bay.

Sometimes people are of an introspective bent and have no problem "sitting down with themselves" and thinking about the totality of their lives. Such thoughts lead inevitably to the question of what you value in your life, what you cherish, what you hold important. Reflecting on the priorities of living leads to thoughts about priorities in dying. My intuition is that most people can come to accept the fact that they must die. But the means of their dying are not so plain and do not rest so comfortably in people's minds. People, I think, fear unrelieved pain, abandonment, and loss of dignity. Where in the past we looked to hospitals for comfort and solace in dying, increasing numbers of people now look at the modern arsenal of medicine with all its high-tech interventions as a threat to dying a good and peaceful death. For the Swansons, the plight of their friend crystallized feelings and thoughts that they had held just one step short of mobilizing themselves to action.

Defining Terms

An advance directive for health care is a written document that may be used as a guide for caregivers in the event that you become unable to express your own wishes relative to the specific options involved in treatment. *Advance directive* is a general inclusive term for a document that seeks to direct future health care for an individual unable to consciously make choices. The term is less familiar to most people than *living will*. Following the Quinlan case in 1976, California became the first state to enact legislation in the area of health-care choices, and living will became very widespread term due to its inherent media appeal. Nonetheless, both terms mean that a person has executed a written expression of the kind of care they wish to receive in the event of accident or illness that leaves them unable to make a competent decision themselves.

By implication, living wills assume that in a conscious, fully competent state you are able and willing to act as your own moral agent. Obviously there is no need for a written document if you are able to think, reflect, and speak for yourself. The question of precisely what is a state of competence can sometimes turn into a knotty psychiatric or legal problem. Because a sick person's state of consciousness may wax and wane, a person may well go in and out of the capacity to make health-care decisions. Likewise, a patient may be competent to make decisions that require minimal exposure to complex treatments and procedures but at the same time be unable to make a decision that would require absorbing a mountain of information (say, for a cardiac transplantation) or that would necessitate the subtle weighing of pros and cons for such a contemplated surgery. As long as the relative nature of the competent state is recognized, assuming too much or too little about a sick person's state of decisionmaking capacity will not unduly paralyze the process.

The other crucial concept that may be useful in guiding care decisions is the term *durable power of attorney*. All states have durable power of attorney provisions that can be used for a wide variety of specific circumstances including designating someone else to make health-care decisions. Like living will legislation, some states have established a statute that describes a specific durable power of attorney instrument for health care. This durable power of attorney is a written document that would legally and formally grant the power to make health-care decisions to another person designated by you only in the event of your incapacity to make such decisions yourself. Typically this person would be a spouse or a close friend. In the event of your serious illness, this person would literally stand in your place and make the decisions you would make if you were able. It is very important that any surrogate decisionmaker you choose know in a detailed and intimate way what you would want in a specific circumstance. The person must know, for example, if you would want to be fed with a stomach tube. Your surrogate must know not only what your general ideas on this subject might be, but must know your mind in a quite concrete and particular way.

States have enacted living-will legislation in all but a few jurisdictions. Other states have acted to achieve legislation spelling out terms for durable power of attorney for health care. Some states have both kinds of legal instruments. It is extremely important to become familiar with the legislative acts that pertain to your state. You should also not assume that your state's legislation may be helpful in all instances with respect to individual treatment decisions. At least two states (Ohio and New York) have set narrow boundaries regarding terminal-care decisions. Given the political contentions around the issue of life-sustaining treatment, it is not surprising that in certain situations a living will or durable power of attorney document will in effect constrict the health-care choices you may have in mind for yourself. Ohio law, for example, specifically excludes the discontinuation of treatment from any person who is *not* terminally ill. The bill also requires artificial fluids and nutrition unless death is "imminent." As we know, death may not come so soon to a person in the persistent vegetative state. You can see that one should not be presumptuous about the laws that relate to health care. You may choose to consult a lawyer or bioethicist who is well versed in these issues. Consumer- and health-lobbying groups may also be very helpful guides about the particularities and peculiarities of your state's laws.

Advantages and Disadvantages

What are the advantages of going through the trouble of drawing up an advance directive for yourself? First of all, the instrument validates in no uncertain terms the principle of autonomy—the idea that you determine what you want in the way of medical care. The old way left many decisions to doctors. They did what they thought was in your interest and for your benefit.

Now we know that the practice of medicine is much too important to be left to doctors. An advance directive makes clear for others just exactly what your interests are.

A second advantage of a living will or durable power of attorney is that its existence will greatly relieve the kind of anxiety your family members would be bound to have should you become seriously ill and unable to make decisions for yourself. Often the shock and sadness of a critical illness will freeze family members in indecision. They will walk around numb and confused about what should be done in regard to your future care. This is exactly what happened with Alice and Bart Swanson's friends following a devastating stroke in their family. A written document or a previously designated proxy will go a long way to dissipate indecision and guilt.

Advance directives also tend to calm the legal liability fears of caregivers. The fact that there might be a specific law that gives a physician immunity from suit in an area of health-care decisions could lessen the desire of the care team to do a lot of unnecessary tests and procedures that might otherwise be done to cover their legal posteriors and to be able to say that they did absolutely everything it was possible to do to save the patient (even things beyond commonsense like resuscitating a patient in the dying stage of terminal cancer). With your written preferences in the medical chart or your surrogate at the bedside, unwanted, uncalled-for treatment is much less apt to occur. In fact, the physician who ignores legal advance directives (either of a statutory or common law nature), risks legal action for violating your right to refuse or to withdraw from a treatment you find unacceptably burdensome.

What about the disadvantages of getting your medical treatment wishes onto a legal document? I believe the risks are few and far outweighed by the benefits. An idea that deserves some thought is the notion that what's down on paper (or in the mind of your surrogate) reflects what you felt *at a certain time in your life* when you drew up and signed the document. People change, as do their ideas about what they want done in particular healthcare situations. Are you the same person today in the intensive care unit critically ill and unconscious as you were seven years ago when you constructed your living will? Have you changed your mind about medical-care directives? Does your thinking about your preferences reflect the latest care and procedures, not to mention outcomes of your illness? The question of the difference between the person you were when you constructed your living will and the person you are at the moment of confronting a difficult choice in the midst of a critical illness is indeed a troubling question in ethics. Very few people can say that they have experienced critical illness and on the basis of that experience are setting out to create a document that reflects the wisdom of such an experience. Therefore, most of us are left to speculate what we might want done in the future regarding critical-care decisions. Advance directives are then entirely a hypothetical exercise. If you were really sick, who knows what you might want? In the context of the crucial moment of decision, who can say what you would want?

Ultimately there is no answer to this dilemma of making decisions in the midst of constant flux. The Greek philosopher Heraclitus, who said that we cannot stick our toe into the same river twice because of the water's constant flow, captured the kind of constant change that every human must bear in mind when thinking about advance directives. All of us change over time. Medical care, as we have seen, radically changes with time. So what we must do is weigh the practical problems of establishing a voice that will carry beyond our own body/mind's ability to speak for itself versus in effect throwing up our hands, casting our fates to the wind, and letting others decide what should be the character and extent of our care in a life-threatening situation where we are unable to act as our own moral agent.

All of this argues for the necessity of periodically renewing and revising the living will instrument. It is not hard to imagine a very problematic set of circumstances where caregivers might have a hard time believing or respecting an out-of-date living will. Family members, too, may have doubts about what you would want done or not done today, irrespective of your written wishes seven years ago, when you may have felt differently about a lot of things.

So living wills are not infinitely flexible, nor can they be expected to cover every contingency and anticipate a person's evolving values. Life is too uncertain, too full of surprises, to be reduced to a few pages of a document. A durable power of attorney is more flexible, but it, too, is not perfect. When we later consider model advance care documents, I will again take up these issues.

The other major consideration in thinking about the possible disadvantages of an advance directive is the argument that we enter a slippery slope when we allow patients to decide if they want to forego life-sustaining treatment. Some people argue that it is the duty of caregivers and hospitals to preserve life at all costs because life is by its nature sacred. But to preserve a biological existence, to keep a collection of organ systems functioning without thinking of the well functioning of a whole person, is to somehow narrow the definition of what it means to be human. And to argue that you cannot exercise some choice in medical treatment that has no benefit other than preserving biological life is somehow to miss the point of why we are all participating in this life journey.

Some who are antagonistic toward living wills also argue that the slippery slope of allowing choice will lead to the legal acceptance of euthanasia. This will happen, opponents say, because respect for life will have eroded. I can point out only two things: 1. Frustrating patient control of life and death health-care decisions feeds the public appetite for more dire measures like physician-assisted suicide and euthanasia. People fear the modern dying process. They want the measure of control that advance directives offer; and 2. Intention makes all the difference in distinguishing between letting die (and thus accepting or surrendering to a disease beyond ultimate human control) and the active taking of life in euthanasia, where the intention is to intervene to end an illness (and a life). Choosing not to prolong dying lacks the ego and arrogance of the act of pretending to control life right up to the end that is implied in suicide or euthanasia.

Life Story

The most interesting story is the one we are in. Who knows what twists of plot or revelations of character await our tale. In the midst of our own life, a narrative unfolds continually. As characters "trapped" in a complex plot, we know only that every story has an end, but we haven't a clue of exactly how our particular story will end. This fact can be tremendously disconcerting. The realization that our life has limits has given artists and philosophers the impetus to imagine and contemplate variations of our common predicament.

As our lives become more and more the sum of the choices we make within our own story, most of us navigate through time with but an occasional glance or a reluctant glimpse toward the end of our days. Sickness—serious sickness that we experience ourselves or through another—is often the sledgehammer that breaks through our persistent illusion that this life can go on indefinitely, one day following another without end. But illness is the rude interruption that opens the door for a larger truth to enter our conscious minds.

If we are to die (an incontrovertible fact beyond our control), can we not at least control the circumstances of our death? Isn't this tempting prospect the real cause behind the movement for patient autonomy that expresses itself in all this talk of living wills. "Living" wills—the very term is provocative. The human will living beyond the body's death! Human ego and pride asserting themselves by spilling out from the grave! Or is this desire for control all a laughable illusion? Can we really control such things? Or is this another human vanity, a product of an age that future historians will say wanted to engineer and plan everything.

Or is the wish for control more a question of fear than of vanity? We humans not only fear death, but probably fear more the possibility of unremitting pain, loneliness, and humiliation. This fear in turn drives a desire to give order to the very disorderly and unpredictable process of dying. We tell stories about death so that we can have some power over it. We share myths that give us the courage to see into the mystery that is death. But our night-sea journey is taken alone. The living will or durable power of attorney we may clutch to our breasts as we near the end of our voyage may provide some people with a measure of comfort and security. Others may sense the irony, the illusion of relying on a human-made plan in confronting the power of life's greatest mystery—death.

Creating a model for dying is the human attempt to control a secret and troubling perplexity by literally giving words to it. The words may be contained in a myth that explains death, in a novel like *Moby Dick* which explores death, or, in the modern instance, in an advance directive that spells out the desired circumstances of passing beyond this life. Literary works and myths are realizations of the secret fears and longings of human beings. The sources are the deep springs of the unconscious, the imagination, and the simple and profound common experience of living. Advance directives, on the other hand, tend toward the rational and the legalistic. The language is cool, detached in tone, objective. It tries to anticipate problems, suggest solutions, give reassurance to misgivings. The completed document partakes of the auras of the lawyer and the analytical philosopher, with a suggestion of a well-meaning state legislator mixed in for good measure.

Considerations in the Advance Directive Document

The limitations of an advance directive for health care notwithstanding, I would still maintain that the execution of this document is worth pursuing. Of course there is the risk of philosophical folly, or just plain skepticism that any legal or quasi-legal document can be equal to the task of willing a certain quality of dying. But the drama of our lives goes on. What also goes on is the power of laws and institutions to affect the lives we are leading. If you do not in some way attempt to have your last days be true to the general tenor of your entire previous life, your last days may resemble whatever the dominant forces of the moment think they should. The power and inertia of the medical colossus will tend to shape your death as it has defined the choices of your medical treatment.

So I think there is a danger in drifting with the ideology and practice of a given time. The risk is not simply folly, or doubt, or pursuing an illusory goal as in, for example, executing a living will. The greater danger of *not* executing a living will is that in effect someone else will if you don't. Again I say, do not underestimate the power of the medical system, with all its riches, technical solutions, and accumulated prestige, to significantly influence, even control, the circumstances of your death. I remind you that these days, four out of five deaths occur in medical institutions.

There are two recent developments that also argue for a proactive stance regarding end-of-life issues. The first is the United States Supreme Court decision in 1990 in the Cruzan case. As I have mentioned, the case concerned a permanently comatose young woman whose parents sued the state of Missouri (Nancy Cruzan was being cared for in a state institution) for the right to disconnect her from daily feedings by means of a stomach tube. The court's decision has many implications for the rights of patients and the rights and responsibilities of surrogate decisionmakers like Nancy Cruzan's parents.

For the first time the Supreme Court validated the general ideas of discontinuing burdensome treatments, including artificial nutrition, in patients in the persistent vegetative state. The court also agreed that previous expressions of a patient's treatment preferences are appropriate instruments for deciding what to do in an end-of-life situation. However, the court did not accept the previously expressed verbal wishes of Nancy Cruzan. Instead, the court demanded a higher standard of advance directive to guide care. The higher standard is a properly executed, per the state law of a given jurisdiction, written advance care document. The court was very eager to take away as much ambiguity and doubt in these matters as it could—thus the very high standard called for by the court. Since Nancy Cruzan was in her late twenties when her devastating automobile accident occurred, she, like most others her age, had not executed an advance directive. But since the

Supreme Court has spoken, it is incumbent on anyone concerned about the issues of dying and appropriate medical care to listen carefully.

The second crucially important development is the Patient Self-Determination Act passed by Congress in 1990. The provisions of the law began to be implemented as of November 1991. Basically the law requires health-care providers—hospitals, nursing homes, health maintenance organizations, home health agencies, etcetera—to maintain a written policy on refusal of treatment and advance directives. Anytime a person is admitted to a hospital, for example, the institution must give the patient information about the basic rights of informed consent as well as the organization's policy on advance directives. The law also provides that the health-care institution provide patients, staff, and community with education about advance directives.

The effect of the patient self-determination act will be a quantum leap in consciousness about living wills and the durable power of attorney. Talk about these instruments will become much more frequent and broad-based. Every patient who enters the medical system will have to at least give cursory attention to the matter of the kind of care preferred in a life-threatening illness or injury. Because the focus on the patient's choice and some of the ideas about care are presented at the point of admission into the system, the declarations of the patient will be duly noted and charted. This kind of official recognition does not necessarily guarantee that preferences will always be respected or that care decisions will always go smoothly, but it is a step toward a standard of care that says it is willing to listen to the voice of the patient. The more widespread and accepted the practice of advance directives becomes, the greater chance that the powers in medicine will listen.

One of the problems in the past has been that the medical

system (and here I'm referring to a wide range of players from physicians to hospital administrators to admissions personnel to paramedics) have failed to even seek out the existence of an advanced directive. I have seen family members in a panic over a stricken parent or spouse call emergency services for an ambulance. Only after calling do they remember that the patient did not desire resuscitation in the event of a cardiac arrest. When they greet the paramedics at the door with this information, it is most often ignored. In the face of an ambiguous situation and without anything in writing, the emergency crew is trained to act in order to save lives. They would rather face the consequences of an inappropriate rescue than stand by and do nothing.

Likewise, when a patient arrives at an emergency room or a hospital for a medical problem, the question of a living will will most often not even come up. I have observed situations where a patient's living will makes it to the medical chart in a doctor's office but does not make it onto the hospital chart when the same patient is hospitalized. I have also noted living wills that are buried in hospital charts and pretty much ignored by all caregivers. In this situation it takes a very assertive patient or family to demand due recognition for the living will. In the context of the fear and shock of serious illness, being assertive is nearly impossible for many patients and their families.

These kinds of situations all argue for the formalized and routine recognition of advance care documents. Imagine if hospitals and nursing homes considered these instruments as important as the insurance information that they so assiduously seek from every patient at the front door. Indeed, loss of Medicare and Medicaid reimbursement is the stick that will face institutions who fail to comply with the provisions of this legislation.

Documents

The paper instrument that you might want to use as an advance care document for yourself may be very philosophical or very legalistic. Let me quote the preface for two documents that might give you some idea of how to approach the important issues to be raised in your reflections about your own life. The first statement is from the American Protestant Health Association:*

> I believe that death is a natural event in the course of human life. Every person has the right to live and die with dignity. I affirm my human right of autonomy which allows me to die my own death within the limits of legal, social and personal factors. I have the right to die with dignity—respected, cared for and loved.
>
> Death consists of more than biological factors. The personal and human processes of life are to be considered along with the biological. I desire that life support systems be used so long as they can aid the continuation of the quality of my personal and biological life.
>
> I consider as unjust the continuation of artificial and mechanical life support systems through expensive medical and technological means when there is no reasonable expectation for my recovery of meaningful personal life. Therefore I am free to refuse such medical treatment which only prolongs my dying.

---

* American Protestant Health Association, 1701 E. Woodfield Rd., Schaumburg, IL 60173.

PLANNING FOR ILLNESS

> In order to avoid the useless prolongation of my dying and the suffering of my loved ones, I am signing a document making known my will regarding my medical treatment in the case of my terminal illness.

Another example of an advance directive preamble is from the group Choice in Dying:*

> Death is as much a reality as birth, growth, maturity and old age. It is the one certainty of life. If the time comes when I can no longer take part in decisions for my own future, let this statement be an expression of my wishes and directions, while I am still of sound mind.
>
> I wish to prevent my assets from being used to unnecessarily prolong my life, so that they may be used instead to benefit others. Also, I wish to avoid the heartache to my loved ones of an extended illness and to avoid additional pain and suffering to myself.
>
> If the situation should arise in which there is no reasonable expectation of my recovery from extreme physical or mental disability, I direct that I be allowed to die and not be kept alive by medications, artificial means or "heroic measure." I do, however, ask that medication be mercifully administered to me to alleviate suffering even though this may shorten my remaining life.
>
> This statement is made after careful consideration and is in accordance with my strong convictions and beliefs. I want

---

* Choice in Dying (formerly Concern for Dying/Society for the Right to Die), 200 Varick St., New York, NY 10014.

the wishes and directions here expressed carried out to the extent permitted by law. Insofar as they are not legally enforceable, I hope that those to whom this will is addressed will regard themselves as morally bound by these provisions. This is my decision—not yours—and is made after careful consideration.

You can see that the flavor of the above examples is personal and philosophical, reflecting in a general way the values a person may wish others to consider in the event of serious illness. You can also see the possibilities for infinite variation in a statement you may wish to write to express your own particular wishes.

Other advance directive documents tend toward impersonal, obtuse, dense legal language to achieve their goals. Mercifully I will not quote from such documents. I will mention only that despite their blandness, such instruments may still be advantageous depending on the state in which you reside. California's and Ohio's Durable Power of Attorney for Health Care are two such documents that residents of these states should at least look at in considering an advance directive. Certainly there is no law that would prevent people from attaching a statement of personal philosophy to such a legal instrument to create a well-balanced total expression.

Before getting into the writing of a model advance directive, it would be well to look at another state's effort to put together a useful document. In Michigan, the state's medical societies, bar association, and hospital association got together to write a Designation of Patient Advocate Form. The document, reprinted in Appendix II, is above all a user-friendly instrument. It is clear and accessible, combining minimal legal language (though it is a legal document in Michigan per Patient Advocate Act, 1990) with specific treatment options. The margins of each page thoughtfully give instructions on how to fill out the form.

I can personally attest that the form has been a hit in my office. I use it both for the person seeking to clarify thinking about future care and as a device to stimulate such thinking. At any rate, the short document is a smashing success in Michigan. Over three quarters of a million copies were distributed in the first four months it was available.

The examples I have cited are the common instruments used by people like yourself to influence the kind of treatment they would want should they become incapacitated. The cited examples by no means cover everything you might want to include in your own document. But they are most representative of the kind of advance directive that people are creating.

I think it would be profitable to spend a little time sketching out some of the goals and potentials that an advance directive for health care can achieve. The "perfect" advance directive I have in mind would be neither too simple nor too complex, too vague in its brevity or too unwieldy in its length. The document would satisfy legal requirements for a particular state, would reflect the lived priorities of its creator, and would both shine in its clarity and be supple enough to bend in the face of an unforeseen circumstance. The ideal advance directive would have qualities of the living will as well as a provision for a surrogate decisionmaker.

No matter how perfect a document you construct for yourself, it is vitally important that the completed document make a prominent debut into the world. What must *not* happen is to place it in a trusted desk drawer at home or in a safety deposit box alongside other valuable papers. An advance directive must circulate! Your spouse, your designated proxy, your children, your doctor, your attorney—all should have a copy of the document and be familiar with your intentions in creating the instrument. Giving these key people a chance to read and discuss your care preferences is a good way not only to spread the word but to further refine and clarify what you want. Their response to your healthcare directives, in the form of questions and comments, will be a good way for you to gauge how effective you are in communicating your choices. And bringing these matters to the forefront at a time when you are physically and mentally sound is an effective means of educating a wide circle of loved ones about your treatment preferences. When and if you become seriously ill and incapacitated, they will remember these previous conversations.

What I would like to do is to attempt an advance directive for health care that would incorporate the features I have described. I will first give you a look at the document, and then walk you through it, section by section, commenting on why things are the way they are. I think the process will be a valuable exercise in the thoughtful creation of such an important document. And on a more personal level, as I go through the process myself, I will be constructing my own advance directive. That's right, even bioethicists can rationalize and procrastinate away getting down to brass tacks and actually creating a concrete directive. I fear the truth is that it is much easier to write about living wills and such, to advise others of the pitfalls of medical-ethical decisions, and to stand above it all with a certain purported clear vision that in reality turns out to be a blind spot. Advance directives are for other people, aren't they? The next time I'm in a roomful of bioethicists, I'll be tempted to ask how many have acted to create an advance directive for themselves.

So here goes my own new and, I hope, improved version of an advance care directive:

PLANNING FOR ILLNESS

Advance Directive For Health Care

SECTION 1: PREAMBLE

I understand that death is part of life. Death is not necessarily an enemy, but ultimately a natural passing from one state to another. I believe that death is both the law of God and the law of Nature, God and Nature in my mind and my experience being intimately bound. The human tendency, on the other hand, is to avoid death and go on living insofar as that is possible. This I also believe. I love the sweetness of life despite the common travails and sorrows that come everyone's way, including my own. But there comes a time to let go, to not prolong the inevitable fate of dying.

This document will attempt to spell out as best I can what I see as parting circumstances—those medical conditions that tend to make impossible the living of a recognizable human life. This is a life where thinking, feeling, experiencing, remembering, reflecting, and relating to other people are not possible. It is a truncated life where there is no more growing and preparing for future concerns and other lives. It is a biological state and not really a human life.

If the time comes when I am no longer competent to make health-care decisions for myself, I wish that the advisories contained in this document will guide my caregivers. I have carefully considered and spent a lifetime of reflecting about the issues that this document addresses. In the event that my fate falls between the lines of this directive, I direct that decisions be made by my wife, who, having accompanied me for most of this long journey, best knows my mind and by the terms of this document possesses legal power of attorney for matters of health care.

SECTION 2: TREATMENT PREFERENCES

Incapacitated States*

	(I) PVS	(II) Mental Incapacity Associated with Illness or Injury	(III) Mental Incapacity Associated with a Terminal Condition
Therapy Choices			
Resuscitation (CPR)	no	M, U, D**	no
Ventilator	no	M, U, D**	no
Dialysis	no	M, U, D**	no
Artificial nutrition	no	M, U, D**	no
Surgery with substantial risk	no	M, U, D**	no
Antibiotics	no	yes	no

M: Maybe. U: Undecided. D: Don't know.

SECTION 3: TERMS DEFINED

Resuscitation: emergency heart and lung treatment with chest compressions, oxygen, drugs, and electroshock in order to restore vital functioning. CPR=cardiopulmonary resuscitation.

Ventilator: a respirator machine that breathes for the lungs when they cannot breathe on their own.

Dialysis: treatment with an artificial kidney machine to cleanse the blood of wastes.

* See pp. 115–16.
** See pp. 116–17.

Artificial nutrition: stomach tube, nasogastric tube, or central venous line for delivering nutrition to persons unable to eat.

Surgery with substantial risk: a procedure with significant chance of death, long-term pain, or disability due to anesthesia, blood loss, infection, or stress on vital organs.

Antibiotics: oral or intravenous medicine designed to fight infection.

SECTION 4: DESCRIPTION OF INCAPACITATED STATES

I. PVS: Persistent vegetative state, or permanent unconsciousness. (See Chapter 3.) A person in the persistent vegetative state is unable to relate to other persons or transact the functions of daily living such as eating or bathing. Only low brain functions such as breathing, heartbeat, and digestion are maintained.

II. Mental Incapacity Associated with Illness or Injury: This is a large category of acute insults to the brain that could result from a head injury, a stroke, meningitis (infection of the lining of the brain), or other trauma. Most often when treatment begins in this category of incapacity, the exact diagnosis may be indeterminate and the prognosis uncertain. Often only extensive medical testing and time will tell the ultimate outcome.

III. Mental Incapacity Associated with a Terminal Condition: Many diseases (especially cancers) that end in death affect the body in such a radical way that disordered thinking, dementia, or unconsciousness may result in addition to fatal damage done, for example, to the lungs, liver, or bowel. Some primary diseases like Alzheimer's affect the brain/

mind directly and ultimately lead not only to severe dementia but to death.

SECTION 5: PROVISOS RELATED TO THERAPY CHOICES

1. I would want resuscitative efforts to be applied as long as my prognosis is uncertain. But if CPR leaves me comatose, I would like to forego further CPR attempts.
2. I see the mechanical ventilator as a temporary bridge to better health and recovery. If I cannot be weaned off the respirator within 90 days, I wish that this therapy be withdrawn and not reinstituted unless a new and remediable acute process intervenes such as a metabolic derangement or a pneumonia. Should I be re-intubated, the 90-day clock would start again.
3. Dialysis as a temporary measure is acceptable. If I should be in a coma state and in need of permanent dialysis, I would not want it. Dialyze me until I'm mentally capable of deciding for myself about treatment of permanent kidney failure.
4. Again I see this treatment as a radical temporary measure to sustain my body during the healing process. If my digestive tract cannot repair itself, I would not want this treatment. If I am comatose but not PVS, I would be willing to go with artificial nutrition for up to 6 months without any sign of improvement in my state of consciousness. I would want to go on for up to one year of this treatment if in the opinion of my surrogate I am making steady progress toward increased mental alertness and functioning. If despite all measures taken on my behalf I have not returned from a coma at the end of one year, I would want all artificial feedings stopped

and comfort measures only by mouth (ice chips, sips of Vernors ginger ale, fruit juices, etc.).

5. The benefits and burdens of any proposed surgery must be weighed by my surrogate. Please, no thought of organ transplantation (other than kidney). Also I want any do not resuscitate order that may appropriately apply to me to remain in effect during and after any surgical procedure.

General Note on Pain Relief: My wish is that I remain as lucid and conscious as possible through the course of a serious illness. However, when pain interrupts and cuts off interaction with the world, I hope that palliative measures will be undertaken on my behalf, including the use of powerful narcotics. Don't spare the horses, please, and don't worry about such untoward side effects like addiction or respiratory depression. If possible, patient controlled analgesia (PCA) would be an excellent solution to many pain problems and most in keeping with respecting my autonomy. In the event I am semiconscious and in apparent discomfort, I would expect aggressive pain relief to be established by my physicians. For state of the art pain therapy, I hope my physicians will be in tune with the latest methods used by hospices to control pain. I wholeheartedly endorse this organization's philosophy as well as practical wisdom in dealing with these matters.

The above choices and provisos in my living will shall be reviewed and appropriately revised or renewed every five years.

SECTION 6: DURABLE POWER OF ATTORNEY FOR HEALTH CARE

(Attach appropriate form per individual state statute.)

In the absence of the relevant state law, attach general power of attorney form specifically naming a surrogate decisionmaker for health care:
I, _____, hereby appoint _____, a competent adult of my own choosing, of _____, _____ to be my attorney in fact to make any and all health-care decisions for me should I become mentally incapacitated to make such decisions for myself. Such decisions shall include but not be limited to choices involving the initiation, withholding, withdrawal, and limitation of any and all treatments, including life-sustaining therapies. My proxy decisionmaker should bear in mind those values I have tried to live and should seek to avoid any therapy that is a significant affront or indignity to these values. In the event the above-named person is unwilling or unable to carry out my wishes or is unavailable, I hereby designate _____, of _____, as my alternate attorney in fact.

My attorney in fact is hereby granted the right to receive information regarding my medical condition, may inspect my medical record, and confer with my physician(s) and other caregivers. I have discussed my living will and the powers and responsibilities of being a proxy decisionmaker with the designees named herein. They understand my treatment preferences and the lifelong values that stand behind my choices.

PLANNING FOR ILLNESS

This power of attorney becomes effective when I can no longer make my own medical decisions and shall not be affected by my disability. I wish the following limits to be placed on the authority of my attorney in fact or alternate: _____
_____
_____ or NO LIMIT

Principal: _____ Date: ____
Witness: _____ Date: ____
Witness: _____ Date: ____
Notary Public:

A Commentary on the Advance Directive Document

My aim was to create an accessible, readily understandable guide with enough specificity to be helpful to my family and caregivers, and enough generality to be flexible in an unforeseen circumstance. I do not think it is possible to plan for every contingency. Nor do I think it is wise to be too vague in expressing treatment preferences.

The preamble gives the reader a sense of the person behind the treatment preferences. It is a chance to reveal one's overall philosophical and religious conception of the issues that the document addresses in more particular, concrete terms.

The length and depth of this introductory section are entirely up to your own discretion. What I think is important is the chance for you in executing an advance directive to express in your own words how you see yourself in relation to possible incapacity and diminishment, and the threat of death. If you want, you can establish a context for the values you are living. Given the very personal nature and wide array of values in our culture, I don't think you should rely on a prepared or "canned" introductory statement such as is commonly used in living-will forms. Since you are unique, I think your statement should reflect this glorious fact.

In contrast to the open-ended and subjective nature of the document's opening, the treatment-preferences section really gets down to brass tacks. Three categories of mentally incapacitated states are presented along with specific choices of therapy. Sections 3 and 4 briefly define and describe the terms used in the treatment-preference grid. You may want to know more about a particular option, say, kidney dialysis. You may want to know the frequency and duration of treatments, life expectancy of a dialysis patient, the physical and psychological side effects of the treatment. To do an adequate job in determining your treatment preference regarding dialysis, you may want to do some research, ask questions of nurses and doctors familiar with this kind of therapy, or even talk to someone currently undergoing dialysis. Only by becoming informed in a very direct way about this possible treatment choice can you come to any reasonable decision about your own choice. So the definitions and descriptions in these sections are a kind of shorthand, really just a beginning in getting to know what you might face in the future.

For the sake of example I have made some choices of my own. Note that what I term Mental Incapacity Associated with Illness or Injury is a very broad category. Treatment decisions here are not often clear cut. Diagnosis may not be sure, prognosis may be uncertain. Therefore in Section 5 I have spelled out certain qualifications with respect to the length and manner of proposed therapies. These personal provisos delineate in more precise terms exactly what I would want. As a further refinement to a simple yes or no choice, which, as we see, is often impossible, these annotated treatment choices may comfortably guide my future caregivers through clouds of uncertainty and ambiguity. Likewise, the intention to revise and recertify the living will every five years is a good method of keeping the document fresh and relevant. Care in doing this assures that there is a meaningful correlation between the living person who created the will and the frozen words on the pages.

The designated durable power of attorney section will vary depending on the state jurisdiction. The model set forth here will work in states that do not have a durable power of attorney for health care statute. I think it is also important to note that you should not think in terms of executing a living will *or* a durable power of attorney instrument. The preferred course is to do *both*. This way, you will not only have a written document to speak on your behalf, but a living advocate as well—someone who can embody your wishes and give some nuanced direction in your mental absence. So I strongly urge you to do both. You will significantly increase your chances of being heard through the tumult and din of a critical illness when it is all too easy to be swept away by the medical system.

Obviously, after all the effort you will have put into your advance care directive, you will want the document to be official and legal. If you are not confident that your instrument conforms to relevant state laws and has been properly executed, by all means consult an attorney. In some states where specific forms are readily available and widely recognized, consulting a lawyer may not be necessary.

So in a typical situation, a husband and a wife, much like Alice and Bart Swanson, would sit down together and talk of these things. A good way to start such a conversation (a conversation which in the larger sense has really been ongoing through the course of a relationship) and get into the particulars of a living will might be for two people to look at a living-will form and let that be the basis of a discussion. Each might fill out a form as he or she thinks the other would like to be cared for. This may produce some surprises. If you have up to this moment avoided being explicit about the kind of medical care you prefer in a critical situation, drafting a will as you think your partner would like it might well unmask assumptions that have no basis in fact. Likewise, your partner will try to gauge what you would want, and depending upon a multitude of factors may or may not be accurate about your own preferences in care. I think this little exercise can be very instructive. It may well serve to open up the discussion of advance care directives to a new level for a couple grappling with this issue.

While writing this chapter I ran into a person who after hearing what I had in mind about living wills and durable powers of attorney said all well and good for that portion of our society which is literate, educated, and interested in more than a passing way in these issues. But, he said, what about the mass of people, the average person who learns about health-care issues from Tom Brokaw, Phil Donahue, or Oprah? Isn't this entire discussion somewhat removed from the average person's ability to deal with these complex problems? In short, he asked, isn't the whole tone and substance of living wills elitist?

My friend has a point. Not every person or every couple would be comfortable or able to discuss all the ideas implied in a living will. Many might not like the form I have offered as a model. Others might feel so powerless and manipulated by the various systems in our culture that they may not trust such an imposing document with all its quasi-legal implications. Still others might sincerely reject on religious grounds any sort of plan for dying or discontinuing life-sustaining treatments. I do recognize the whole gamut of possible suspicion and objection that advance directives might engender in the minds of many people. But I would still contend that we all share a part of the same life together. Our common human fate—death—links us one to the other. Together we experience the common fears and pains of illness, the same dark hard knot in the pit of our stomach in facing the very disturbing realizations of the soul. This kind of philosophical knowing combined with the double-edged sword of modern medicine (it can prolong dying as well as living) creates in many the need to reassert the human measure when evaluating technological medicine. In a way, people seek to mark territory in creating a living will. They seek to define the boundaries of the human, the limits of a life, and the appropriate map that gives direction toward a proper dying. This is powerful stuff, this thing that pulls us toward a fitting end. And there may well be degrees of understanding and articulateness that would distinguish a simple living-will document from a more sophisticated one. But both speak of a common human fate.

I believe that significant numbers of people in recent years have experienced the technological dying of a loved one, the carrying on of life beyond hope or common sense. Most do not wish this for themselves. This kind of experience is an important impetus behind advance directives. Now, the form of such a medical directive may well have to take on a multitude of appearances. There will be those who desire a short, sweet, and simple form describing their choices for care. Others will be attracted to more complex, complicated advance directives that spell out in some detail exactly what is desired. Still other documents may fall between these two possibilities. My point is that all sincere and legal forms should be honored and respected. In fact, we should celebrate the possible diversity of advance directives and the unique voices and lives that go into their formation and elaboration.

We all should also seek to make a compact with the person

who will be given the task of speaking for us when we are unable to say what we want. This proxy must know something of the values we have tried to live. Not only should this person know us in the general sense, but should have specific, concrete knowledge of our own treatment choices. This requires a long and close relationship, where something of the inner core has been revealed to another. When we have accomplished this relationship of comfort and trust, health-care decisions in the incapacitated state are much more likely to be congruent with our lifelong values. I would note only that the voice that may represent you can be helpful no matter what your position in life, no matter your level of sophistication in medical decisionmaking.

CHAPTER 5

Growing Older: Ethical Issues in Aging

What shall I do with this absurdity—
O heart, O troubled heart—this caricature,
Decrepit age that has been tied to me
As to a dog's tail?
      —W. B. Yeats

So teach us to number our days that we may get a heart of wisdom.
      —Psalms 90:12

Introduction

  The question the great Irish writer posed reminds me of many office visits with older patients. After a follow-up exam for a chronic condition such as arthritis or diabetes, a patient might feel moved to comment along the lines that "growing old sure isn't easy," or "nobody told me that being old would feel like this," or "Doc, I'm beginning to feel like a grandfather clock slowly winding down." Usually such remarks are offered in an offhand or humorous tone. I try to receive them as graciously and sensitively as possible. But what is striking is the evident need to talk about the aging process, to articulate the feelings of what it's like to come up against the ultimate human limit—a lifespan numbered in years.

The poet's question about what one should do with the knowledge that each of us will have the absurd decrepitude of old age pinned to our own tails is a fitting question to contemplate. What does it all mean? How does one handle the aging process with a degree of grace, acceptance, and dignity? What health-care decisions are important to think about relevant to old age? What are some of the choices, some of the pitfalls in dealing with the medical system so as to improve your chances of having a sense of accomplishment and fulfillment in your final stage in life?

The statistics that describe our aging society have become at least vaguely familiar to almost every American who reads or who watches the nightly news. Ours is a culture that is beginning to reap the consequences of greatly improved hygiene and high-tech medicine. It's no secret that people are living longer. But the paradox of this success is that people now live longer and therefore have more opportunity to develop one or many serious acute medical problems and an almost certainty of developing a chronic condition that requires regular care. It seems that life indeed does wind down.

Like the law of entropy that physicists say governs the universe, our own bodily universes seem bound by the same law. Things fall apart. Living things decay. Perfect order degenerates into random chaos. Gradually and surely, living things go back to a more elemental, a more disorganized form. Furthermore, like the boundaries to life itself that first come into view sometime in childhood, the process of entropy is remorseless and inevitable.

I do not mean to paint a dark picture. In fact, because our lives have these hard limits does not mean that there is no hope or joy in fully living our days. But we must not stick our heads in the sand. To savor our time, even the time toward the end of our lives, we must face the realities of the temporariness of our time on this earth.

The later years of life are often referred to as the time of twilight, the time of low light and lengthening shadows. But sometimes the light at the end of the day can be a light that illuminates reality in a way not seen at any other time of day. Filmmakers and photographers call this special time of luminous light the "magic hour." Impressionist painters were also well aware of the potential of the late light of day to reveal the essence of a landscape or a building. They knew that the sun's course in its late stages could reveal more than the sun of high and bright noon. Late day, late life, can be a time to open up to the world in a new way. Potentially it can be a time where it can be said that we'll be as wise as we'll ever be. Rank ambition, planning careers, achieving—all can be laid aside in old age. Finally there is a time to relish the fruits of our labors and to watch the passing parade with new eyes, and to ponder just what it all means.

The Aging Society

It is instructive to compare age statistics from the start of the twentieth century to the present time. The figures tend to dramatize the gray wave that is upon our culture and underscores some of the problems of making life extension one of the goals of our medical system.

By 1990 there was an eightfold increase in the number of persons in the United States aged sixty-five or older as compared to 1900. Whereas at the start of the century the group of people aged sixty-five or older constituted just over four percent of the population, by 1990 they represented twelve percent of the population. By 2035 the same group will make up twenty-two to twenty-seven percent of the total number of Americans. By 1990 fully eighty-five percent of all females born in the U.S. reached age sixty-five. This compares to the one in twenty chance of reaching age sixty-five that faced eighteenth- and nineteenth-century Americans of both sexes.

But today the fastest-growing population group is the men and women aged eighty-five and over. This group has shown a tremendous twenty-one-fold increase in the ninety years of this century. The implications of this explosive growth in the ratio of older people to working-age people are extremely troublesome. Whereas in 1900 there were seven elderly for every one hundred working people, today the ratio is more like twenty elderly for every one hundred working people. Estimates project that this ratio of old to working will increase by the year 2020 to twenty-nine to one hundred. How can a society afford to support the burdens of its own success?

With increased longevity goes the increased chance of developing both acute and chronic illness. With increasing age, statistics show a dramatic increase in doctor visits, in-hospital days, and nursing home admissions. Lifesaving therapies may create opportunities for further episodes that are life-threatening. Then the inevitable chronic diseases move in and establish lifelong residence in aging and weakened bodies. In short, we see more and more people living longer and feeling worse.

The question is how long can we continue as a society to dodge some of the issues around debility and death? The sheer and disturbing economics of the situation are leading some to ask philosophical questions. For example, in 1960, fifteen percent of the federal budget went to entitlement programs that benefitted the elderly. By 1990 more than thirty percent of federal moneys was spent for the same purpose. Projections for the future are so awesome that the question must be asked: Can we afford to support the indefinite prolongation of life to the detriment of other worthy priorities like the education of the young, housing for the needy, and a decent environment free of noxious threats? Is not one of the tasks of the old to in good time step aside? When vitality wanes and ripeness turns to withering, the old have an opportunity to pass on their cultural achievements and legacy by first forming a link with the past, creating a perspective of times past for the young, and then, in due course, as part of the nature of things, move on and make way.

This is not to suggest a callous attitude toward the old, nor do I mean in any way to suggest that the old should be shoved toward death's door. But surely each of us in time must pass on. When and how we do it are on a personal level one of the central questions of our existence. On a societal level the question is also important, for how we approach those in the shadows and failing light of late day is a crucial measure of what a society values.

Something of what I'm talking about is symbolically captured in a Greek burial custom that is still practiced today. A loaf of bread is placed on the coffin and together, bread and body, are lowered into the ground. The fundamental idea that the bread symbolizes is imparted in the words of the priest: The earth which nourished you, now will consume you.

Ethical Issues in Aging

It was the American literary critic Malcolm Cowley who observed that we first start growing old in other people's eyes; later, slowly, we come to share other people's judgment. What does this new status of being old imply? Growing old first suggests the waning of physical and intellectual powers, though this is not universally true of all aged people, nor does it happen quite the same way, if at all, in each individual. But for most people the passing of time into the sixth and seventh decades of life is marked by a certain creakiness in the joints, a diminishment in stamina, a less steady step, and, for some, a memory that has blurred or extinguished certain details of experience.

With the lessening of powers come the threats to one's integrity as a person. Independence that has been earned, exercised, and exalted in a culture that venerates the individual above all suddenly can come under threat. Dependency I would guess strikes most Americans as a negatively charged word. It means having to depend on others—family, friends, nurses, doctors—for some of the basic needs of daily living. Being dependent also means being at the mercy of various institutions—the Social Security Administration, Medicare, medical institutions, maybe even the local bus company.

With the coming of dependency, which may arrive suddenly, as in the case of a stroke, or gradually, as in progressively crippling arthritis, the erosion of personal autonomy accelerates. The lack of extended families, the generational bridge, if you will, makes the loss of autonomy all the more stark and disconcerting. The fact that we live in a youth-obsessed culture that does not honor the traditional or the old as repositories of wisdom contributes to the feeling that old means useless. In America in the last half of the twentieth century, useless items are cast off.

How are you to contend with this process of reduction? How are you to maximize your freedom, autonomy, and powers as you journey through the final years of your life? What specific ethical issues will you encounter? The following sections will attempt to illuminate these questions.

GROWING OLDER: ETHICAL ISSUES IN AGING

Long-Term Care

In the recent literature about care of the aging, the phrase *long-term care* enjoys a currency. Discussions about reforming the American health-care system, papers detailing problems in old age insurance, commissions charged with coming up with practical recommendations about the problems of aging, all use the phrase *long-term care* in preference to the more familiar and chilling term *nursing home*. I would grant that there is more to long-term care than what is implied by a nursing home alone and that long-term care is a more global concept than what the average person understands a nursing home to be. Still, there is no denying the negative connotations of nursing homes. To many, the image is of a place to warehouse the old, a dirty place with poor care, bad smells, and little freedom. In short, a place where no one would want to be. How often have we all heard sentiments expressed along the lines "Promise me that you won't ever put me in a nursing home" or "I'd rather die than go to a nursing home."

In fact, nursing homes have done much to reform the abuses of the 1950s and 1960s. They not only become a "home for life" for many of their residents, but also a temporary stop on the rehabilitation trail for those who require short-term help during the recovery and restorative process. Before considering some of the problems that remain in nursing homes, it might be well to consider some alternative arrangements that you might want to consider.

Obviously the goal is to remain functioning in the world in which you have been living for as long as possible without compromising your health and safety. Like everyone else, you want to preserve the ability to come and go as you please, take care of your daily needs, like cooking, dressing, and bathing, as well as meet the demands of caring for particular health problems. At some point you may need help with some or all of these tasks. The best help, and the most common, is extended by the watchful and caring intervention of family members. Though they probably would not live in the same household, some relatives might live close by and be willing to take on some care responsibilities. Their help might be as simple as looking in on you periodically, driving you to the doctor's office, or tilling up your garden space in the spring.

Given the far-flung nature of American families, sometimes it is nearly impossible to get help from relatives. Often friendly neighbors will take up the slack in these situations. I see this often in my practice. I never fail to be amazed at the generosity of caring—one individual for another—though they are virtual strangers with no long-term ties of blood or association. They are just thoughtful neighbors and their simple caring blunts somewhat the merciless cult of American individualism.

There are other sources of help for the elderly homebound. Home-care nurse visits have become increasingly common over the last several years. In fact, for the past five years the number of home visits has expanded at a rate of twenty percent annually. The schedule and needs for visits are usually determined by the team of nurses, social workers, and doctors who are caring for a given patient. A relatively short-term schedule of visits might be arranged following a surgery. The nurse will visit the home, assess the patient, her environment, and the specific health problems at hand. The nurse might typically do a dressing change, administer intravenous medications, or teach the patient about a diabetic regimen of care. In short, home health extends the medical system into the comfortable and familiar place of residence.

A number of other resources are available for the person confined to the home. They range from voluntary programs like Meals on Wheels to Medicare-funded services such as physical therapy. Home health aides are also available on a regular basis for purposes such as maintaining personal hygiene. Other home care can be arranged in many areas to accomplish such things as shopping or doing housework. And don't forget the community at large which can provide a youngster to mow the lawn or shovel the snow or a local hairdresser to come into the home or the minister or priest to visit on a regular basis.

In addition to the wealth of helpful services available to come into the home, there are other alternative living arrangements to consider when the burden of living alone and independently becomes too great. The popularity of the "grandmother house" has caught the imagination of many in recent years. Typically this is a separate living quarters constructed for an elderly relative. It may in rural areas be a free-standing one-bedroom cabin or bungalow built next to the home of a son or daughter. In a suburban locale the grandmother house may take the form of a separate wing built onto the main house. In more urban locations, the elderly may live in an attached apartment or in a part of a larger apartment with their own bedroom, bath, and sitting room. In every variation of this sort of living arrangement, the chance for achieving a balance of privacy and community, space and closeness, is maximized. Meals (perhaps most commonly the evening meal given the practices of most American families) may be taken in common, perhaps most typically three generations together, or on other occasions the family may choose to not be together. In times of an elder's disability or illness, the option is there for closer scrutiny and direct care to encourage healing. This type of living arrangement is extremely flexible, limited only by the imagination of the families involved. And it is much, much less expensive than a nursing home. One can imagine in the future what tax credits would do to encourage this kind of alternative living arrangement.

One other option that may appeal to the elderly who care neither for the nursing home or retaining their independent home or apartment is an aggregate living arrangement. This type of cooperative group living takes several forms. One form is an apartment building or complex devoted entirely to the old. Individual apartments are provided, together with the positive features that might be seen in a nursing home: skilled nursing services, the option of taking meals in a common eating area; cultural programming such as concerts and movies; great attention to wheelchair access and creating a generally safe environment; help with the tasks of shopping and transportation; emergency medical access.

Other forms of elder cooperative living arrangements might be more loosely organized with a range of opportunities and services that would appeal to a wide range of physical capacities. Everything from walking trails to golf courses to swimming pools to lawn bowling might be offered to maintain physical tone. Many such places for the elderly also take steps to ensure that the mental edge is kept honed. They sponsor lectures, field trips, and, most interestingly, short courses resembling college classes and often taught by local university professors. The topics range from Shakespeare to ecology to philosophy. What better way to keep your edge and test the wisdom of your age?

Nursing Homes

For most, nursing homes represent a place of last resort for care of aging people who are unable to totally look after themselves. Families almost invariably seek nursing home care reluctantly. Usually it is after a period of trying to marshal resources together to care for a parent or grandparent who is steadily and progressively failing. To say the least, the decision is emotionally wrenching and sometimes ethically troubling. It is a decision often filled with guilt. But sometimes it is also a release from the anger and frustration of a long period of attempting to care for an elder who has increasingly demonstrated an inability to care for himself. Often this inability to successfully deal with the tasks of daily living is the major reason for seeking care in a nursing home.

Other times the onset of dementia is the trigger that leads to nursing-home placement. Dementia is the more or less sustained but sometimes reversible state of mind in which there is an observable decline in intellectual functioning. It is fleeting memory, especially short term memory; it is a certain dulled or obtunded state of consciousness that can be caused by any number of illnesses that affect the brain, of which Alzheimer's disease is the most common. Fully two-thirds of nursing-home residents are to some extent demented. This state of mind knows many variations. Some people wax and wane in and out of dementia with windows of clarity that may be frequent or infrequent. Others seem to constantly live in another realm, some apparently happily, others not. Some demented persons are aware of the defect in their intellectual performance, others are not. Given the wide diversity of presentation of the demented state, it is wise to assume that every person with significant mental deficits can understand and communicate at some time or at some level. Staying as reality-based as possible with the demented person, being open to the possibility of communication, and giving clues and prompts that may stimulate communication are all necessary to prevent the extreme isolation of dementia.

Marked physical disability or failing health that requires skilled nursing care are also admission tickets to a nursing home in the absence of other feasible alternatives. The onset of urinary or fecal incontinence is a common trigger to seek professional care. Inability to walk or frequent falling down with resulting bone fractures also is a reason for many to seek the help of an institution.

I am reminded of a case presented to our medical school class Problems of Aging where the teacher described a patient. The facts of the case portrayed a female who appeared her stated age and could neither speak nor comprehend the spoken word. She babbled incoherently for hours, was disoriented, unable to recognize her caregivers, but was seemingly responsive to her own name. The professor went on to describe that the patient tended to disregard her physical appearance and made no effort to participate in her own care. He stated that she needed to be clothed, fed, and bathed by others. Since she had no teeth, her food was pureed. She was incontinent of urine and stool and tended to drool incessantly. She slept erratically and for no apparent reason would sometimes scream or go into crying fits.

The professor then asked the medical students how they would feel about caring for such a person. It was not hard to elicit replies that spoke of the inherent frustration and lack of satisfaction in being involved with this person's care. Something inside all of us recoils at the thought of having to be involved in such a sorry situation.

But then, quite unexpectedly, the professor told us that he really enjoyed taking care of this person, and that he did it all the time. He then opened his wallet and passed around a photograph of the person described in the "case"—his four-month-old daughter!

It was an effective way of making his point and probably

helped change the perspective of many medical students regarding caring for the aging. Despite the obvious differences in caring for the very old as opposed to the very young, there still exists the similarities of helplessness and dependence. It is also instructive to reflect on how the start of our voyage through life seems to resemble the end of our journey. Is it traveling full circle back to where we began? What is this sometimes utter dependence on others a preparation for? As our worldly powers weaken, is there any compensating gain?

Institutional Issues

Being admitted to a nursing home, or "placed," as the current lingo would have it, forces one to experience what is known as the *total institution*. In a sense, one's entire life is taken over—managed, regulated, and controlled for one's own good. The total institution, of course, runs directly counter to the American dream of self-reliant, independent individualism. Nursing homes surely run against the American cultural grain. This partially explains their unattractiveness to the average citizen. Moving into a nursing home is more than a simple change of address, and most often it is different from being admitted to a hospital. Make no mistake about it, nursing-home residence represents a significant change in life.

In the United States over 2.3 million persons reside in over 19,500 nursing homes. Given their relative longevity, three-quarters of the residents are female. The annual costs of nursing-home care is more than it costs to support a student at Harvard. It is more than the annual expense of incarceration at America's most secure prisons. Depending on the quality of the facility and its services and the amenities offered, nursing homes cost from twenty-six to fifty thousand dollars per year. Approximately one-half of this expense is borne by patients and their families, forty-four percent by Medicaid, and the balance from private insurance.

Since there is no Medicare benefit for long-term care, most families find that their resources are quickly depleted by the burdensome costs of nursing-home services. In fact, of those single elderly who acquire Medicaid coverage, over ninety percent "spend down" in the first year. This required exhausting of personal assets is one of the most devastating and humiliating aspects of nursing-home care for many families. The message from the larger culture seems to be that if you can't do anything, you can't have anything. And remember, the message is coming from a society that supports sophisticated technology, drugs, and techniques to extend life. But once one reaches a certain point—the intersection of old age, disability, and poverty—the floor seems to drop out from under the person who had been counted previously as a medical success story.

One way many families are fighting this kind of unsavory treatment of the old is by organizing, lobbying, and pushing for meaningful change in the American system of health care. Others are consulting attorneys about legal ways of preventing hard-earned assets from falling victim to spend-down provisions. By planning ahead and executing the right series of gifts and trusts, it is possible to legally prevent assets from being used up. Some think this kind of action damages the already precarious system of care for the old by forcing the expenditure of dollars and perhaps depriving the truly needy from access to Medicaid nursing-home care. Others believe the strategy is not only legal, but a political device that forces society to take a close look at the problem and perhaps reform the system as the cracks in its foundation become more and more apparent.

So what are your chances of someday ending up in a nursing home? Grossly stated, if you live beyond sixty-five years of age, your chances of one day using a nursing home are one in four. This figure, of course, includes short recuperative stays. Surprisingly, over seventy percent of persons who need nursing-home services are eventually discharged from the facility with a median duration of stay of less than three months. Looking at overall use of nursing-home care, there is cause for some optimism. Before age seventy-five, only one percent of the population will reside in a nursing home at any given time. This compares to twenty-two and a half percent of the population over age eighty-five, who live in nursing homes. With the total population tilting in the direction of the old old, you can see the coming vast demand for nursing-home services. But the good news remains that up to age seventy-five, you have a ninety-nine percent chance of maintaining an independent or semi-independent (requiring some help) life-style. Until age eighty-five, your chances of remaining self-sufficient are over ninety-three percent. The figures demonstrate that in general nursing homes are inhabited by the debilitated very old or by persons needing services for a short-term recuperative period.

Privacy Issues

Since nursing homes so take over the lives of their residents and are responsible for all aspects of care, it is no wonder that communal living arrangements tend to erode away lifelong habits of privacy. The adjustment for you, or for a family member, indeed for anyone, must reach down into the very hidden spaces of a person. One way of conceiving of nursing homes is the image of a refuge or a retreat from the welter of a modern industrial-information society. Nursing homes are places for the very aged to seek a respite from the incessant demands of such a world. As such, it is important to evaluate a facility as to how sensitive they are in allowing residents to retain some semblance of their past private lives.

It is a question that has both an attitudinal as well as an architectural aspect. Is the staff alert to the necessary psychological withdrawal from the world that residents may be seeking? Is the policy and practice of the institution to grant a large degree of privacy to residents if they so choose? Or is being alone somehow seen as pathological or antisocial? Does the physical plant allow both the flowering of communal life through common facilities for recreation and fellowship as well as private sanctums where residents can be quietly alone?

Do residents of a given nursing home have freedom of association? This means the institutional endorsement to be with others of their choosing, when and where they like. Ultimately it means private association. Sometimes it might mean intimate association. Does the institution, in short, give the residents enough space—space understood as both physical environment and the immaterial realm where a person's autonomy is played out? Or does the home have a repressive, very controlled air about it? Sometimes the latter attitude is rationalized as a means to ensure the health and safety of residents.

Nursing-home residents should have the right to choose their own roommates. They should at the very minimum have the right to not be housed in the same room with someone who regularly disturbs and upsets them. In addition, the nursing home should have in place some mechanism whereby disputes with roommates or with staff are aired and settled with the involvement and due consideration of the residents themselves.

The key element in evaluating a home for possible use by an

elderly relative is to consider the overall tone of the establishment. Ask residents how they like it. Ask their families for their impression of the place. Involve the elder, if possible, in the process of evaluation. Talk to staff members you see working amid the patients. What is their general attitude as you observe them going about their daily tasks? How far are they willing to go to serve the needs and desires of prospective residents who may not fit the mold of the average nursing-home resident? And finally the ultimate question regarding problems with privacy: Will they respect what remains of a person's autonomy and will the institution permit a degree of a resident's spirit and personality to run counter to how they would like all of their residents to be?

Restraints

Nursing homes often have the ambience of a clinic. That is, the aura of medicines and nurses and patient charts and treatments pervades the atmosphere of a home. But unlike a hospital, which has as its primary goal the diagnoses and treatment of sickness or injury, a nursing home is often a permanent home for the self, a place where one is taken care of in light of an incapacity to perform many of the tasks of daily living. In a very real sense, nursing homes provide care for diminished selves—persons who have suffered the loss of some vital capacity. The geriatric self that resides in a long-term care facility is a self whose very core as an adult person comes under threat.

One of the principal threats that old persons face is the sudden and astounding loss of freedom. And remember the freedom to move about where one chooses, the freedom to eat what and where and when one chooses, the freedom, in short, to be and to do—these are lifelong habits ingrained in the Western tradition. There is nothing so surprising as losing something you might have taken for granted for years on end. But the loss of freedom is really a paradox. Yes, there is a loss. But there is also a potential gain in that an elderly person may be moving from a dangerous, crumbling environment to one of concern and care. But to benefit from the caring concern of the nursing home milieu, one's frailty and steadily decreasing powers must yield still further and confront the reality of less freedom.

A central moral question facing caregivers is how far to go in restraining freedom for the good of the residents. For example, what if anything should be done about the nursing-home resident who tends to wander? What about the resident who tends to fall (a life-threatening circumstance given that fractured hips are extremely disabling and often lethal)? What should be done about the resident who keeps his roommate awake with long torrents of screams and verbal abuse? And finally, what about the resident who occasionally physically strikes out at other residents or staff members?

Restraints applied to nursing-home residents are of two general varieties: mechanical restraints and behavior-modifying drugs —the so-called chemical straitjackets. Mechanical restraints include cloth devices for the arms and chest that restrict movement, bedrails, or special "geri-chairs" that control free movement. Drugs that affect the mind and emotions by directly acting on neurotransmitters in the brain itself are known as psychotropic drugs. These drugs may be antidepressants, tranquilizers, or antipsychotic agents. As a group, they have profound powers for effecting human behavior. But in a nursing-home setting, their potential for harm is at least as great as their potential for good.

The prevalence of using restraints in nursing homes in the United States is a very slippery statistic to come by. Estimates of the use of mechanical restraints ranges from twenty-five to eighty-five percent of residents. Psychotropic drug use by nursing-home elderly is somewhere in the vicinity of twenty percent in most studies. In practice, the use of mind-altering drugs is a factor likely to prompt the use of mechanical restraints given that fifty-five percent of residents' behavior needing modification was treated by dual controls. It is clear that the use of restraints varies widely from nursing home to nursing home, from country to country. Some U.S. nursing homes are very reluctant to use restraints. Likewise, in Great Britain and Sweden restraints are used only in a small fraction of the instances they are employed here.

Why do nursing homes restrain their residents? There is always the legal liability issue that drives administrators to restrict the probability of harm to their charges. The most common reasons cited for using restraints in one study of fifty-five nursing homes were: unsteadiness of gait, disruptive or agitated behavior, and wandering by residents. Nursing homes often feel caught between the desire to provide safe care in an understaffed home while at the same time complying with the maze of government regulations in providing such care. They feel trapped in the seeming necessity of restricting their residents in order to prevent harm.

But recently several articles in the bioethics literature have challenged some of the underlying assumptions about geriatric care. Indeed, some commentators have questioned both the effectiveness of using restraints and the ethics of restricting nursing-home residents' freedom.

These writers have argued that not only is there no evidence that restraints prevent injuries such as fractures resulting from falls, but that restraints themselves are a cause of significant care and comfort problems. Some gerontologists argue that the number of falls is no less in nursing homes employing mechanical restraints than it is in nursing homes that do not use restraints, or among the homebound elderly. They point out that using restraints often leads to the formation of bedsores, loss of muscle tone, incontinence, dulled affect and sociability, and, in the case of falls, more serious injuries. Up to two-thirds of injuries from falling out of bed occur in patients attempting to climb over elevated bedrails.

Critics of psychotropic drug use in nursing homes cite a study done in 1990 which demonstrated that approximately fifty percent of the nursing-home patients who were being treated with these kinds of drugs did not have a diagnosis on their charts that would justify this kind of treatment. Often the use of these powerful drugs seems to proceed from the argument of expediency rather than from any rational scientific basis. Furthermore, little attention is paid to the problem of informed consent. Recently adopted federal regulations that apply to Medicare- and Medicaid-certified nursing homes require that the use of these types of drugs be justified by indications documented on the resident's chart.

Gerontologists (scholars in the field of aging studies), geritricians (health-care professionals working with the elderly), government regulators, and most nursing-home administrators support the concept of promoting the least restrictive environment possible for residents. Ideally this kind of environment would support autonomy in the face of frailty, disability, and, ultimately, the coming of death. Individual differences among residents would not only be respected, but celebrated as part of the diversity of humankind. The sense of an elderly person's self should whenever possible be enhanced specifically by maximizing an individual's choices. This working out of a person's last years of autonomy requires that caregivers be sensitive to what it means to have failing powers. This often means simply not interfering with what residents want to do and with creating an atmosphere that is pliable enough to bend to individuals' quirks and differences.

In evaluating a nursing home on behalf of a loved one, it is important to keep these principles in mind. One means of deciding about the appropriateness of a given care setting is to judge just how imaginative the administrators and caregivers are in creating a caring environment. For example, have alternatives to restraints been adequately considered?

Beds that are very low to the floor eliminate the need for bedrails. Electronic wristbands that set off an alarm if a resident should attempt to wander off by exiting any of the institution's doors are a good alternative to tying a resident down. Likewise, increased staffing may lessen dangers to residents. There is almost no end to the possible development of gadgets, safety padding, and other measures to make the lives of seniors more comfortable and less restrictive. Perhaps if we as a society can apply the same will to create a safe and supportive geriatric environment as we have done in building space environments for astronauts, we will have gone a long way in meeting some of the long-term health needs of our older citizens.

There are also the more subtle psychological dimensions of nursing-home care. How much of life in a nursing home is rigid, even prisonlike in its routines? Can residents sleep in if they wish? Can they skip meals? Can they prepare simple snacks in their rooms with a microwave oven, for example? Can they have private conversations, person to person, or on the phone? Do residents have access to the outdoors? Can they leave the facility and visit friends and relatives anytime they wish? The answers to these questions will reveal much about the tenor of life within a given home. In fact, this kind of evaluation might reveal if the prospective place of residence for your relative resembles in any way a "home," or is merely a "facility" or an "institution."

The Driving Issue

Another interesting issue for the elderly is the privilege of driving an automobile. For most adults in most locales, driving an automobile is an essential ingredient in being able to negotiate the daily chores of modern American life such as shopping or going to the post office. To the disadvantage of our society, most Americans do not have a public transportation alternative for such tasks. True to the American grain, we instead rely on individual motor vehicles to get us where we want to go. If a person is unable to drive a car, he or she is at a considerable disadvantage at surviving independently in our present-day culture.

As aging accentuates our gradually declining physical powers, nowhere is this better seen than in driving a car. With decreased visual and hearing acuity and decreased muscular coordination and reaction time, the multiple tasks of perception, reflex action, and judgment involved in driving can become troublesome for some older drivers. Some elderly drivers quickly become aware of their own declining driving abilities either through self-observation or as a result of the observations of family and friends. They see the potential dangers and readily give up their licenses. Others are oblivious of their own deficits and often go right on driving despite, in some cases, a record of frequent accidents. Sometimes it takes a horrific accident involving serious injury or death before they are persuaded to give up driving. Almost all state licensing renewals are mere formalities involving neither a driving test nor a medical exam for relicensure of drivers beyond a certain age. Nor do automobile insurance companies require their older policy holders to in any way prove their continuing driving competence.

GROWING OLDER: ETHICAL ISSUES IN AGING

The ethical problem is the classic one involving the rights and duties of individuals versus the good of the community. No one wants to discriminate against an older driver solely on the basis of age. On the other hand, no one would like to see the elderly killing themselves in cars or causing the death of innocent others as a result of incompetent driving. Since depriving a person of freedom of movement is no small matter, can a way be found that would protect the common good as well as individual liberty with respect to operating a motor vehicle? In practical terms, this is an exceedingly difficult balance to achieve. But with efforts from three different sources, it might be possible to accomplish a workable balance.

First, the families of elderly drivers should keep themselves well apprised of the current driving skills of their elders. They should not hesitate to offer feedback in as sensitive a way as possible. They should never back down from their honest assessments and expressions of concern. In extreme cases of denial and after demonstrated endangerment of their elderly loved one's life and those of others, family members might want to move in concert to prevent a disaster. I have heard of cases where family members have arranged for car keys to be "lost" or cars to become mysteriously disabled.

Physicians and home health nurses may also have a role to play in evaluating and counseling older drivers. They can offer advice and cautions about the effects of prescription drugs on the ability to drive. They can offer medical advice about how certain conditions can lessen the proficiency of a driver. They may refer drivers who need help to professionals who can supply a device such as a hearing aid or an automotive aid that might make a particular vehicle safer or easier to drive. Medical people also might be very effective in limiting the kind and amount of driving an elderly person could actually do. For example, it might be reasonable at some point to advise against night driving, or driving on high-traffic expressways or congested city streets, or taking extended trips, or driving in foul weather. But at the same time, driving to town on a local road to get groceries or to visit grandchildren might be an acceptable way for certain elders to maintain limited driving skills.

And finally, various organizations that support safe driving can aim programs at the older segment of the population. Such programs as Mature Driving, sponsored by the American Association of Retired Persons, addresses the issues of declining vision and hearing with an eight-hour classroom course that attempts to build on old skills while developing specific strategies for such diverse problems as handling right-of-way situations, decreased reaction times, and driving under adverse conditions. Senior citizen centers, wellness clinics, state agencies, and insurance companies could all become involved in such efforts that not only would serve the elderly but the public as well.

Medical Care and Surgery in Old Age

Deciding about health-care issues is a problem for every elderly person regardless of his or her particular living situation. As a general rule and in agreement with common sense, the older one gets, the more likely and the more intensely will a person need medical services. This is true of significant chronic problems, for example vision and hearing difficulties or joint pains, as well as for major acute episodes requiring hospitalization such as heart attacks and cancer treatment. Critical choices in therapy that may involve life and death can at least be partially addressed with the use of advance directives. Less imposing or threatening health problems also have the potential to create dilemmas in care choices.

One such area where the elderly must be particularly wary is surgery. Surgery can be life-sustaining and can alleviate significant health problems, such as an inflamed gallbladder or a broken hip. No one can argue about the great contribution that the surgeon makes to relieving distress and curing some diseases. But as an elderly person, one must approach surgery with a certain degree of wariness. For the surgeon's scalpel is the proverbial double-edged sword. When used appropriately and with great caution as to the risks and benefits for a specific patient, the scalpel can make the cut that cures. When used inappropriately and without due concern for the long-term good of the patient, the surgeon's scalpel can be an instrument that promises more than it can deliver and that blinds both the practitioner and the patient to potential and underestimated harms.

Among doctors, surgeons are a breed unto themselves. In Great Britain, surgeons are even addressed differently from medical doctors. They are called mister (and presumably Ms. or Mrs.) instead of doctor. Surgeons are action-oriented. They care very much about short-term results. "Don't just do something, stand there" is a wry piece of advice probably invented by nonsurgeons to poke fun at the surgeon's propensity for immediate and direct action.

Surgery has been described by writer and former surgeon Richard Selzer as a priesthood. It is a vocation with a harsh initiation (long years of training, weeks of sleepless nights), rituals, special vestments, arcane language ("Hand me that mosquito!"), and a cabinet full of special instruments to enter the human body. In realizing the spiritual aspects of the body ("The flesh is the spirit thickened"), Selzer also acknowledges the limitations of surgery. He points out that though the surgeon may know perfectly the landscape of the brain, he hasn't the slightest idea how a thought is formed.

So it is well to remember the mind-set of the typical American surgeon, for sooner or later you will probably need his opinion or his skills. To know that he or she has a tendency to see health problems and solutions in mechanistic terms is to prepare oneself for surgery with open eyes. In my experience with patients I have been struck by how easily people are persuaded to accept the advice of surgeons with hardly a question or a demur. Seemingly, they readily, almost eagerly, follow the surgeon's advice. Is this because they do not know what questions to ask of a proposed operation? Are they awed or cowed by the profession of the knife? Or perhaps are their own personalities much like the surgeon they consult—both embodiments of the American ideal—rugged individualists who want quick results without undue questions or equivocations, without the pretense of soft-headed reflection? In short, are the American patient and the American surgeon in many cases a perfect match?

Still, not all people approach surgery in the same way. I remember a middle-aged women whom I had diagnosed with breast cancer. She needed an urgent surgical consultation for a life-threatening disease which as we know also can have terrible psychological consequences in regard to a woman's body image. So I always considered discussing the various options for breast cancer treatment a very sensitive matter. But this particular women not only took the news well and later readily agreed to a mastectomy, she seemed concerned about only one thing: When could she get back to her Wednesday night bowling league? How long would she be out of action? How would the mastectomy affect her bowling form? This woman went easily to surgery.

I once saw a man who hated to go to doctors. An independent woodsman and trapper, the man had successfully avoided doctors for over thirty years until at age fifty-six his daughter and son-in-law brought him in to see me with severe abdominal pain and bloody stools. Only very reluctantly did Clete agree to blood tests and X rays. When a huge bowel cancer was found, he seemed so terrified of going to a surgeon that his family literally had to pack him into their pickup truck and cart him off for the consultation. Though surgery was advised, Clete never seriously considered going under the knife. A mixture of fear, denial, and pessimism about his own body and the ability of surgeon's to heal it caused him to withdraw to his cabin to spend his remaining few months of life.

The third type of response to the need for seeing a surgeon is the skeptical approach. Being suspicious about the need for surgery, cautious about accepting any one surgeon's opinion, asking multiple, detailed questions about a proposed operation—all of this drives most surgeons crazy. But I think this is the preferred method.

Asking the Right Questions

The wisdom of seeking second, and even third, surgical opinions has been demonstrated. Insurance companies gladly pay for these additional opinions because they know that the more opinions on the medical chart, the more likely a costly surgery will *not* be undertaken. One study demonstrated that eighty-four percent of persons who had at first been advised to undergo bypass surgery by their primary-care physician and cardiac surgeon were persuaded to continue medical therapy for their heart disease after seeking a second opinion. The group was followed for more than twenty-seven months and had no fatalities, and presumably an acceptable quality of life through this period. Clearly this study and others raise the question of whether surgical intervention in a disease process is overused.

Another study that looked at coronary artery bypass graft (CABG) surgery at multiple hospitals examined the criteria for the surgery as it was stated on patient charts and compared these indications to a list of 488 possible indications for bypass surgery developed by a national panel of experts. The study found that thirty percent of the surgeries were performed for "equivocal" reasons, fourteen percent for inappropriate reasons. Only fifty-six percent of the surgeries were done with a clearly appropriate rationale.

So imagine that your internist or family practitioner has counseled you to seek a surgical opinion regarding, say, the advisability of undergoing cardiac bypass surgery, a procedure performed approximately 250,000 times each year in the United States. He arranges appointments with two surgeons from different groups whom you find acceptable. How should you prepare for the surgeons' evaluations?

First, you may want to talk to patients who have had the same procedure and are about the same age as yourself. Your physician or network of friends probably could get you in contact with the right persons. Ask them about their experience of the surgery. Were there any unanticipated problems? What was their level of pain? Have they had any significant benefit from their surgery? If the same circumstances applied in their case, would they agree to have the surgery done again? Never underestimate the wisdom of experience. This way of knowing about cardiac bypass surgery can be crucial not only regarding your own decision, but in generating the questions that will be the basis of your decision.

When seeing your surgical consultant, try to be open, prepared, cordial, and skeptical of everything he might say. Do not under any circumstances allow yourself to be rushed through your evaluation process. Bring your spouse or a friend to the interview. Write out your questions before you arrive at the surgeon's office. Your companion should try to position himself between the surgeon and the door of the examination room. This will make it less likely that the busy doctor will bolt the room before all of your questions are answered. If the surgeon is evasive or if he is unwilling to engage in a real dialogue about your case, cross this person off your list and have your primary-care physician arrange an alternative evaluation.

What are some key questions to ask? You can begin by focusing on the need for the proposed surgery. Has the surgical profession developed a consensus as to the indications for the contemplated surgery? Are there any articles or books suitable for the layperson on the topic of cardiac bypass surgery? Are there nonsurgical alternatives? If surgery is necessary, what about waiting six months or a year? Where will the surgery be performed? Who will perform the surgery? (Remember that in teaching hospitals, residents often do the actual surgery under the supervision of their mentors. You have the right to know and to consent to surgery only if it is to be done by the surgeon of your choice.) What is the hospital's record in regard to morbidity and mortality with respect to cardiac bypass surgery? In other words, what are the statistics regarding complications and death after cardiac bypass surgery at this particular institution? How do these results compare to other hospitals that you name?

It is also appropriate to question the surgeon as to his professional qualifications to do the surgery. Where did he train? How long has he been doing cardiac bypass surgery? How frequently does he operate? (Within limits, the more frequently a surgeon performs a given procedure, the more adept he or she and the rest of the care team become at anticipating problems, mastering technique, and assuring good results.) What is the surgeon's personal record in regard to morbidity and mortality for this procedure? How does this compare with national statistics?

The next thing to consider in selecting a surgeon is whether the physician involved has any financial incentives to perform surgery other than the customary professional fee. Does the surgeon own all or part of a free-standing surgical center? Though cardiac bypass surgery is far too complex to be performed in such a facility, nonetheless the question will smoke out the entrepreneurial operator. Cautionary flags should instantly fly if you suspect that your surgeon looks upon his professional craft as a business. It's only a small step then for him to regard you more as an opportunity than a patient. The present post-Reagan era has resulted in a considerable shift on the part of many physicians from the professional to the business mode. Beware of this tendency in any physician you see.

One of the surgical specialties where the capitalistic spirit is particularly enthusiastic is the field of ophthalmology. Hundreds of thousands of cataract extractions are performed yearly in the United States. In fact, the procedure is reimbursed by more Medicaid dollars than any other single operation. So-called "cataract cowboys" are physicians who set up eye factories for production-line cataract surgeries. Often these entrepreneurs advertise this surgery as "free" and promise extravagant benefits. Sometimes these operators will offer free eye exams and free transportation to the eye clinic. Their target, of course, is the rapidly growing elderly segment of the population. Some of these physicians make over a million dollars a year. The criteria they use to justify surgery are loose, somewhat subjective, and self-serving. One patient had her cataract removed because of a problem with "glare."

So if you perceive a problem, or even a potential problem regarding a conflict of interest in your physician, I think the best advice is to back out of the relationship. Self-referral to a physician-owned enterprise—be it a surgicenter or a lab, or a CAT scan or MRI facility—invites a split vision of you as a patient. This kind of arrangement where the physician operates a practice like a business also encourages overtreatment and overuse of medical technology. At a minimum, physicians should as a matter of course disclose any interest they may have in a profit-making venture connected in any way to their medical practice. If this is done, patients will at least have some choice as to whether they should continue their relationship with this physician. The judgment must be made as to what is paramount in the physician's practice—the doctor's self-interest or concern for the welfare of the patient.

Surgical Statistics

Given the astounding fact that there are over thirty-five million surgical procedures performed in the United States every year (most are minor outpatient procedures), it is no wonder that each person in the country has about a one in ten chance of having surgery done in any given year. Surgery is estimated to account for the majority of hospital admissions and more than half the annual cost of health care.

In order, the major surgeries performed in the United States yearly are cesarean section (800,000), hysterectomy (673,000), dilation and curettage of the uterus (632,000), cataract extraction (630,000), tubal ligation (568,000), tonsillectomy and adenoidectomy (478,000). The figures are based on 1986 information and consequently the present numbers would be different. However, the figures give some inkling about trends and just where all the surgical energy is directed. Curiously, a whole lot of surgery is aimed at the reproductive organs of women. There is fully four times as much surgery done on female genitalia as on male genitalia, despite the extraordinary number of operations done on the overly exuberant or cancerous prostate glands of aging males. Between the ages of thirty-five and forty-four, women in the United States face a two percent risk *every* year of having their uterus surgically removed.

These statistics provide fuel for many feminist fires and should give pause to every surgeon as well as every woman. In no area of surgery is the seeking of a second opinion more necessary. Studies have shown that such factors as socioeconomic status, hospital ownership, payment source, and volume of obstetrical services independently affect the rate of gynecological surgery. Teaching hospitals with resident physicians, high-volume services, and the presence of health insurance all tend to increase the utilization of surgical services.

Another factor that affects the rate of a given surgery in a population is geography. Many studies have noted wide variation in the number of specific surgeries per hundred thousand residents in a given locale. Common procedures such as cardiac catheterization, upper GI endoscopy, and carotid endarterectomy vary tremendously from one part of a state or region and another. For example, you are twice as likely to undergo cardiac bypass surgery if you live in New Haven, Connecticut, than if you live in Boston. However, your chances of undergoing a carotid endarterectomy in Boston is twice what it would be in New Haven. Many confounding and paradoxical factors influence a given region's rate of surgery. It is not entirely clear why there is so much variation. Some say the presence of many surgeons in a given specialty will boost the rate of surgery in their area of service. The argument is that first patients with clear indications for a given operation are treated; then persons with less clear indications ("equivocal") are drawn into the surgical system as the number of clearly appropriate patients dwindles; finally increasing numbers of inappropriate patients are offered surgical services. Some policy analysts claim that the only way to control unnecessary surgery is to limit the number of surgeons or to severely restrict a technology, such as a cardiac catheterization lab, which makes a specific surgery possible. Other studies argue that variations in practice are not due to inappropriate indications for medical procedures. Rather, the problem may be with differences in disease incidence, cultural and social perceptions about care, or differences in referral patterns. Suffice it to say that there are many unanswered questions in the geographic distribution of medical and surgical care.

Summing Up

Facing major surgery is a serious question at any age. For an older person the prospect raises even more disturbing questions and doubts. For the elderly the balance of perceived risks and benefits that a given surgery may present seem oftentimes to tilt away from benefit and toward greater risks.

Everyone who contemplates serious surgery must come face-to-face with uncertainty. There are frequently no hard answers to questions, only responses cast in terms of probabilities. Surgery also causes you to see any procedure in terms of human fallibility. First there is the vulnerable patient in need of an intervention to heal a failing or broken body. This is very basic. Human bodies eventually fail. In ceasing to function at a previous and comfortable level, you may seek out another human being called a surgeon to repair damage and restore functioning. But this is a person too bound by an absence of perfect knowledge, by uncertainty, and marked with the human sign of fallibility.

One consideration about any surgery that seeks to prolong life is the possibility that increased longevity could increase your quotient of misery. The misery would flow from pain of the surgery itself, a potentially prolonged and exasperating recovery period, exposure to multiple complications that risk further disability and even death, and an ultimate surgical outcome that may have as much pain and suffering connected with it as the original problem that motivated you to seek a surgical solution. One patient who was dying of liver failure wrote: "There are worse things than dying too young. One of them is dying too old." The kind of modern "death by a thousand qualifications" may be a fate worse than the kind of death most people imagine for themselves. It was the French philosopher Montaigne who described a more wholesome relationship among sickness, aging, and death:

> I notice that in proportion as I sink into sickness, I naturally enter into a certain disdain for life. I find that I have much more trouble digesting this resolution when I am in health than when I have a fever. Inasmuch as I no longer cling so hard to the good things of life when I begin to lose the use and pleasure of them, I come to view death with much less frightened eyes. This makes me hope that the farther I get from life and the nearer to death, the more easily I shall accept the exchange. . . . But when we are led by Nature's hand down a gentle and virtually imperceptible slope, bit by bit, one step at a time, she rolls us into this wretched state and makes us familiar with it; so that we find no shock when

youth dies within us, which in essence and in truth is a harder death than the complete death of a languishing life or the death of old age; inasmuch as the leap is not so cruel from a painful life as from a sweet and flourishing life to a grievous and painful one.*

Montaigne's wisdom suggests that being old requires the development of certain virtues. To be disposed toward seeking right thought and right action may allow one to see death in its widest context as the natural completion of a life. The following short list of virtues for aging is by no means comprehensive or limiting. It is only a beginning at sketching the powers of human character that might make aging a more decent and honorable process.

When you age you first need courage to face loss, pain, and uncertainty. You also need humility to counter the arrogance and illusion of power that we might think we have over life. Aging also demands the cultivation of simplicity—the ability to travel light, avoiding the weight of complexity and complication. Getting older requires patience and steadfastness; slowly and steadily the days go, inviting an attitude that can wait for small moments to savor. Ripening to old age also requires a certain resignation to the ground facts of the universe; an acceptance of the knowledge of Aeschylus that what must happen will happen. Humor is also a virtue to serve one's spirit well as a lightness, an antidote to the spell of dull gray grimness the world sometimes casts. And finally the virtue of detachment allows you the paradoxical frame of mind that acknowledges that you are not only in and of this

---

* Michel Montaigne, "That to Philosophize Is to Learn to Die," in *The Complete Essays of Michel Montaigne*, trans. Donald M. Frame, Stanford, CA: Stanford University Press, 1965, p. 63.

world, but somehow also apart and beyond the things of matter and time.

Daniel Callahan, bioethicist and philosopher, noted in one of his books that we must learn to distinguish tragedy, outrage, and sadness in thinking about wise human ends. He said:

> It is a tragedy when life ends prematurely even though it is possible to save that life, and when old age is full of burdens even though resources are available to relieve them. It is an outrage when, through selfishness, discrimination, or culpable indifference, the elderly are denied what they need and deserve. But it is only a sadness, an ineradicable part of life itself, when after a long and full life a person ages and dies in a society that has cherished and supported that person through the various stages of life. It is wise to want to banish the tragedy and outrage, but not the sadness.*

---

* Daniel Callahan, *Setting Limits: Medical Goals in an Aging Society*, Simon and Schuster, New York, 1987, p. 204.

CHAPTER 6

Tapping Ethics Resources

"All professions are conspiracies against the laity."
—George Bernard Shaw

Being Hospitalized

One of the worst aspects of serious illness is the feeling of helplessness that seems to envelop not only the sick person but everyone close to the patient as well. Serious illness or injury can strike suddenly, cutting off a person from the familiar patterns and routines of daily living. Hospitalization can be viewed as the ultimate interruption. No one plans for it or wants it, save those few who see the hospital as a respite or refuge from a rougher world. Only dire medical necessity can persuade the average person to give up the comforts of home for the regimentation, lack of privacy, and feeling of powerlessness that are so identified with hospitalization. Truly only rancorous pain, dread of death, or the threat of disability can persuade many a sick person to accede to their doctor's wishes and enter the hospital.

If in addition to the physical and emotional trauma of illness one must wrestle with an ethical dilemma associated with the illness, the feeling of helplessness is compounded. Where can one turn for advice? What resources are out there and how can one tap them in order to make headway toward a solution of a practical problem?

Prudent Choices

The aim of this chapter is to tour the ethics resources that are available to facilitate decisionmaking. The particular strengths and uses of a given person or book or program will be discussed. The goal is to help create a better-informed patient and family so that the burden of ethical decisionmaking is not quite so onerous. With more information comes the chance for greater knowledge. And with a greater knowledge about a particular issue or treatment option comes the greater chance of achieving the ultimate goal of ethics—a wise and prudent choice.

The satisfaction of the prudent, informed choice, given the often-excruciating alternatives in clinical crunches, is the realization that all that could be done, philosophically and ethically speaking, was indeed done. Decisions made on the basis of too little information or in a process that was conceptually inadequate may later bring haunting memories and bitter regret. Poor decisions, that is, decisions about care that do not leave the heart at rest, can be minimized with due consideration and knowledgeable reflection. When choices are made with some degree of openness and confidence, regardless of the outcome of a clinical problem, all parties—patient, family, and caregivers—are blessed with the sense of having done the right thing.

TAPPING ETHICS RESOURCES

No ethical decision can ever be "perfect" because human knowledge, concern, and judgment have never attained the ideal of perfection. The human fate is to live in an imperfect, morally ambiguous universe. In the moral forest where we find ourselves living, we all try to avoid becoming lost, falling into a morass, or becoming prey to the dangerous beasts that hide in the depths. We do the best we can. By being better informed about an ethical issue, we might be able to do better still.

Allies for Ethics

DOCTORS

The doctor-patient relationship arises out of mutual trust, develops with exchanges of honesty, and proceeds to better healing through shared responsibility in decisionmaking. Or such is the ideal. A doctor you can confide in, respect, and trust. A patient who is honest, forthright, and willing to share responsibility for health.

I believe there is a deep craving in the general public for physicians who somehow evoke a feeling for how medicine was in another age. The avuncular old doctor who answers to "Doc," is available anytime, practices alone, is totally devoted to his patients, makes home visits, does everything himself without referring to some cold and expensive specialist, is someone you can easily talk to, is liked even by kids, delivers babies at home, and still charges only ten bucks for an office call. This portrait is a fantasy. Parts of it were no doubt true at one time, but megamedicine—large-scale group practices with advanced technologies available onsite and a corporate/bureaucratic structure that emulates other successful entrepreneurs of the service sector of the economy—has dramatically altered the shape and feel of receiving care in the 1990s as compared to 1940.

The changes have serious implications for trust and honesty in the doctor-patient relationship. In a simpler age, medically speaking, ethics was also simple and straightforward. As a patient, one assumed your physician's ethical competence and proceeded on that basis. With the modern erosions of trust brought on partly by forces larger than medicine itself, including, as I mentioned, corporate organization of medicine, rapid technical advances, consumerist demands from patients, and a more demanding legal accountability for medical actions, there has been a decline in the public estimation of the medical profession. This has created problems as diverse as a decline in the pool of medical school applicants to a less trusting, more contentious relationship between patients and doctors.

There is no time more crucial for the communication and mutual respect pathways to be open for the patient and the practitioner than with the advent of a serious illness. This is often the time of hard choices and ethical squeezes. It is a time for sharing and trust so that the best possible decisions about matters of life and death can be made. For the patient it is a time of great need, a time when every ally of healing is needed to understand the ramifications of personal affliction. For the physician, too, it is a time when trust and openness in dealing with a disease process are essential in order to achieve the best care possible.

So how can one regard the physician as a possible resource in making ethical clinical decisions? Obviously the better the previous relationship with a given physician, the more potential there is to have a smooth and productive relationship through the course of a serious illness. But what about the common situation where a patient may find himself under the care of a new and totally unknown doctor. This would typically occur after an acute

TAPPING ETHICS RESOURCES

heart attack when care might be directed by a cardiologist in a cardiac intensive care unit. What can this physician offer in the realm of ethical decisionmaking?

The first useful thing the cardiologist can do, beyond supervising medical care, is to provide technical expertise. Look upon the cardiologist as a purveyor of information and a source of knowledge about your disease. What is the extent of damage to your heart? What further invasive tests and procedures will he recommend? What will be their possible benefit? What are the statistical chances of living longer and feeling better with and without bypass surgery? How will these heart medications affect my life? What changes does he recommend in my way of living that will be better for my heart?

For these and other questions, the cardiologist can provide answers that will have a direct bearing on decisions that may come up in the near or distant future. Intrinsic to the role of physician is that of the teacher. And again, by becoming more informed the chance of an ethical ambush is considerably lessened.

The physician, in this case the cardiologist, can also play a role as quarterback of the care team. With this leadership role the cardiologist can consult and deliver other expert help to your bedside. Perhaps an occupational therapist to develop a cardiac rehabilitation program, a dietician to review habits and make recommendations, or access to an ethics committee to help resolve some ethical dilemma that could arise. Look upon your physician, even the relatively unfamiliar specialist, as a person who can be the key to accessing a whole range of potentially helpful persons. Remember that physicians possess the political clout within a hospital that can get things done. And remember that you are employing the physician in order to get things done on your behalf.

The physician who takes an interest in caring as well as curing brings the great advantage of clinical experience to any morally troubling aspect of treatment. The cardiologist, for example, has seen hundreds of similar cases to yours throughout training and practice. This provides a beginning point to determine how your own case is both similar to and different from the hundreds that have come before. Combining this clinical perspective with a true regard for what the patient may or may not prefer forms a powerful amalgam in clarifying biomedical choices.

A word about the Hippocratic oath—the oath that all physicians swear, usually at their graduation ceremony. As cynicism and suspicion about the means and ends of medicine have grown, so has skepticism about any possible use served by an ancient oath, often referred to, reflecting our times, as the "hypocritic" oath. Yet there are doctors and scholars who would argue that the oath of Hippocrates contains the core ideals of medical conduct, including respect for the dignity of patients, moderation in the pursuit of treatment, and modesty, generosity, and self-restraint in the practice of the profession of healing.

Most physicians, I would guess, do not think very much about the specific interpretations of the oath. However, almost all physicians are aware of the ethos of medicine—those core ethical values that guide the healer toward healing with due regard for the patient and the society of which they both are a part—and this awareness, reinforced through years of training, does indeed take root. Most physicians try to put the interests of the patient first. In fact, many treatment dilemmas occur when the physician forgets this paramount concern and pursues a course of treatment that through arrogance and ignorance is a path that does not regard the autonomy of the patient but is the doctor's will alone.

Becoming familiar with the Hippocratic oath might be a good way for patients to enter into the ethical ideals of their physicians. Although it is unlikely to provide solutions to concrete ethical problems, it is a useful expression of the ethical tenor of medicine. As such, what it has to say may hint at a virtue in need of development in a medical-ethical dilemma or the oath may suggest the basis for a discussion with your physician.

NURSES

No one is closer to the patient in a hospital stay than the nurses who daily labor at the bedside. Being with the patient for eight to twelve hours a day, nurses more clearly understand the suffering a patient is going through than any other caregiver. Nurses know what distress is. They know patient frustration. A patient's vulnerability and helplessness are plain to see for the bedside nurse. Where the doctor sees the patient for a few minutes a day, the nurse spends long hours providing care and comfort in addition to crucial medical interventions.

The nurse is also in a unique position to observe the family of the ill. Observing daily visits, seeing interaction among family members, talking with family about their concerns—all this contributes to nursing's intimate perspective on a family in crisis. The nurse is often the first person to notice a problem in family dynamics that could express itself later when a critical care decision must be made.

Nurses are also the most supportive persons that patients meet during their hospitalization. It is not surprising, then, to see extraordinary bonding occur between nurses and patients in the course of a long hospitalization. Nurses stand up for their patients. They often represent the patient's interest in care conferences with doctors and other caregivers. In standing up for their patients' best interests, nurses stand with and help give meaning to the suffering they witness. Make no mistake about it. It is the sympathetic heart and the helping hand of the nurse that is most often the most memorable aspect of care for seriously ill patients.

Sometimes the nurse is compromised in her ability to provide optimum care. Imagine a situation where the nurse is sympathetic to a patient's desire to limit care, for example in the case of a patient who does not want cardiopulmonary resuscitation to be carried out in the event his heart stops. The patient, the family, and the nurse all agree on the appropriateness of this decision due to the grave circumstances of the case. But suppose the physician wants all-out aggressive therapy and will not write a DNR order on the chart. Needless to say, the nurse would find herself in a very delicate situation. How far should she go in advocating the patient's position? How far can she realistically go in persuading or cajoling on behalf of the patient before she risks alienating the physician? This is not an uncommon situation in the politics of rendering care.

In a situation where an ethical choice has to be made by a patient and family, the nurse is a good source of straight, down-to-earth medical information, and like the doctor is a point of access to other resources in the hospital that may be helpful. A nurse in an intensive care unit is tuned to the rising and falling of patient hopes, is experienced with the practical realities of decisions to withdraw or withhold treatment, and can read the body's signs as well as anyone.

In my experience I have seen the bedside nurse as the key person who made the difference between a case turning out well and falling apart badly. The observations and judgments of nurses close to a case are ignored at great peril.

Families who have a nurse as a member or a friend are also at an advantage. I recall a case where the seventy-two-year-old patriarch of a large Greek family was lucky enough to have a daughter-in-law who was a nurse. The man had just suffered a massive stroke five weeks earlier, followed by complications with his lungs and kidneys. It was a terribly complicated medical picture. Due to the stroke, the patient himself was not capable of making decisions. The daughter-in-law served as a conduit between the wife of the patient and other family members and the medical team which consisted of four different doctors at that point (one each for brain, heart, lungs, and kidneys). She was able to cut through the medical jargon and ask pointed questions about the prognosis of her father-in-law. She educated the family to the basic physiology of the disease process and clued them in about the medical technologies (respirator and dialysis) that were being employed. She also took on the role as spokesperson for the family. This was tremendously helpful and avoided the confusion of multiple voices repeating questions or hearing the crux of what the doctors were saying in totally different ways. She was in effect a clinical interpreter of events.

As the case dragged on and the wife was beginning to be overwhelmed by the loss of her husband and the guilt of not being able to prevent her husband's life from being sustained artificially when the medical team had proposed a gastrostomy tube, the wife remembered her husband's words before his stroke. It was during a hospitalization about a year and a half previously. He told her: "No tubes. Let me go peacefully if it comes to that." Now she was faced with the choice between betraying her husband's wishes and allowing her husband to die by refusing more treatment. All of this was tremendously burdensome, troubling, and confusing. The resolve to refuse the feeding tube was galvanized by the nurse in the family. She demanded and got a conference with all her father-in-law's doctors and explained the family's position. Next she requested some informal consultation with the hospital ethics committee to recapitulate the issues as the family saw them.

In the end she was instrumental in carrying through the patient's wishes. As an experienced nurse, she knew that aggressive therapy, including cardiopulmonary resuscitation, had no place in her father-in-law's care plan. The medical crisis for the family which had become an ethical crisis as well came to a resolution that all the family members could accept. Mr. Petrokis died peacefully within a week.

FRIENDS

Friends represent a lifetime of mutual trust and caring. It would be unlikely that a friendship would have flourished for any appreciable length of time without enduring, clear communication. In knowing another person, the superficial aspects of personality and character fall away, revealing something of the heart of the other.

Friends also represent a range of skills, talents, accomplishments, and powers. They can give good advice, even-handed counsel, or can be a good sounding board. They know something of your moods and habits and predispositions. Friends know what you value and what you abhor. They can appreciate, as few others can, the unfolding story of your life. They can offer a perspective that is impossible to get from anyone else.

In the course of a serious illness, friends will be around. They may offer the usual sympathies and you will feel refreshed by their attentions. If the illness should require the kind of troubling decision that we see again and again in medicine, think of close friends as potential resources for coming to grips with difficult choices. The social-worker friend, the lawyer friend, the neurologist friend—they all may be able to offer professional advice as well that bears on the problem at hand. If you should find yourself caught in a bioethical crunch, view the web of connections among your friends as a network of possible clarity and support.

ETHICIST

Ethicists are a new breed of academic and clinical animal. Rising to a kind of prominence with the coming of bioethics to the mainstream of the medical encounter, bioethicists have come from many different backgrounds. Many are refugees from what used to be called moral philosophy. These people somehow or other wandered in or were invited into the clinic to observe the real world of ethical choices. Most liked the invigoration of adding practical or applied ethics to their theoretical repertoire.

Other ethicists came to the field through theology, the ministry, or religious studies. They, too, found the medical clinic a fascinating interplay of ethical forces and moral conundrums. And many were experienced in dealing with the personal dramas of individuals in crisis. Others were more attuned to academic arguments, scholarship, and teaching.

Persons with experience in medicine, nursing, social work, or other allied health fields have also found their way into the bioethics movement. Previous work in dealing with specific health problems and observing patients through the course of an illness mark the clinically experienced practitioner of bioethics.

So people come to biomedical ethics from widely varying backgrounds. How does one specifically prepare for the work of counseling others about ethical questions? One way is to seek an academic degree in a philosophy or medical humanities department. These programs usually, but not always, have a clinical component designed to provide exposure to the medical and nursing context.

Training programs in clinical ethics take six months to two

years. These programs offer opportunities for research and writing, designing ethics education programs, working with institutional ethics committees, and, most important, an apprenticelike experience in the real world of consultative bioethics usually carried on in a very large medical center.

Broadly speaking, there are two distinct breeds of bioethicist. One is based in a medical school and is academically oriented, which is to say his or her primary activity is teaching and research in health-care ethics. Often such ethicists also serve on hospital ethics committees, lead regional and national conferences and seminars, and occasionally consult on individual ethics cases as they may occur in the university hospital.

The second kind of ethicist is exclusively hospital based and concerned not only with case consultations but with working on hospital ethics policies such as a do not resuscitate policy. The hospital ethicist is also deeply involved in the ethics education activities of the medical center as they relate to medical and nursing staff, resident physicians, administration, and hospital ethics committees. The ethicist in effect becomes the principal hospital resource for the myriad issues that daily come to the forefront as values relate to health care.

A third model for the ethicist is the independent consultant. This mode of doing ethics is by providing educational, policy review, and consultative services to hospitals and health-care training programs. This allows medium-size institutions to meet their needs in ethics without committing themselves to hiring a full-time person.

If a patient or family becomes embroiled in an ethical dilemma that seems to resist a solution, the services of an ethicist could be very advantageous. Obtaining this kind of help would be as easy as asking the attending physician or the nurse for some time with an ethics consultant.

TAPPING ETHICS RESOURCES

Consultants in ethics operate from a number of different model bases. Some claim an expertise in ethics. Declaring oneself an expert in ethics is of course very problematical. It's like setting oneself up on a moral pedestal and could be misconstrued as an arrogant and presumptuous stance to take. Other ethicists are careful to claim only limited expertise. They would say they are experts at the *process* of ethical problem-solving and counsel individuals and families so that they can examine their own values and arrive at a decision consistent with those values and the values of the medical culture. To be fair, I know of no ethicist, whether claiming expertise or not, who renders moral opinions and seeks to push his or her own views on a patient or family.

It is interesting to note how much of an aura the word *bioethics* conjures up in some people's minds. It has been my experience that most people I encounter are simply mystified and dumbfounded by what the word *bioethics* could possibly mean. A colleague of mine, a Canadian, would regularly cross the border in her overladen van, tell the customs officer she was a graduate student, and then invariably be interrogated. Sometimes she could not cross the border without a search of her vehicle. Then one time she hit upon the idea of giving a slightly different response to the custom officer's query about the nature of her business in the United States. "I'm doing a fellowship in bioethics in the U.S." The customs officer paused, repeated the word *bioethics* to himself, and then quickly waved the van through the gate. It was as if she had said, "I am an emissary of the good. I study ethics. Both the Pope and the Queen of England endorse what I am doing."

An alternative model for the ethics consultant involves the roles of educator and facilitator. Instead of wearing the cloak of an expert, the ethicist attempts to learn the facts of a case and provides relevant information and knowledge to the patient, family, and caregivers. The ethicist tries to clarify the issues, answer questions, and cut through the ambiguity and complexity of many ethical issues. One ethicist has suggested that the role of the consultant is comparable to a midwife who educates, supports, encourages, and stands by as the principal parties attempt to deliver their own moral resolution. This model of consultation has the merit of recognizing the moral sense that most persons have accrued through a lifetime of moral decisionmaking. The consult is designed so that the parties can come to some realization about the right and the good of a given problem.

Engaging the services of an ethicist does not necessarily help solve every clinical problem. What happens, for example, when two trusted consultants disagree about what is the right action to take? What is an ethicist to do if a patient is intent on a decision that clearly violates a societal consensus? What if, for example, the parents of a Down syndrome baby refuse to consider corrective surgery to repair their infant's esophagus? This kind of case often arises. Too often these kinds of questions are almost reflexively pitched into the court system for resolution.

Making difficult moral choices is not easy. Among themselves, at their meetings and in their journals, ethicists are a contentious and argumentative lot. Like everyone else, they don't necessarily have the answer. And like everyone else, their glory is in the integrity of their search for a right answer.

ETHICS COMMITTEES

A clear trend of the last twenty years has been the establishment of hospital ethics committees in American hospitals. While only five percent of hospitals had committees in 1970, today it is estimated that more than sixty percent of hospitals have one or more ethics committees. In the very large medical centers there could be an ethics committee for each unit that has the history or expectation of treating problematical cases. Neonatal intensive care units as well as adult critical units are two examples of the kinds of places in a hospital that might well have an organized and functioning ethics committee.

In some centers the hospital ethics committee, sometimes termed the institutional ethics committee, is exclusively concerned with the tasks of ethics education in the hospital and policy setting and review as this relates to ethical issues. Individual case consulting, however, is a job taken on by many ethics committees, especially after the committee members have matured with more and more experience as well as greater acceptance by the medical, nursing, and patient constituencies of a hospital community. Cases are most often brought to the attention of the committee by either patients, their families, or, most commonly, the medical staff. Practice varies, but in some institutions only doctors can bring cases to the attention of the ethics committee. In other hospitals, cases are referred by social workers, nurses, or other parties who believe they have a substantial ethical problem.

The first task of the committee is to decide whether a given problem falls within the domain of ethics. Some questions may deal with personnel problems, labor relations, religious disputes, psychiatric problems, or legal claims. Clearly, not every issue with a moral shading belongs on the agenda of an ethics committee. Other forums, be they legal or religious or personal counseling, are often far more productive in resolving problems. However, there are issues, such as racism and sexism, that some ethics committees will take on if it can be demonstrated that patient care is being adversely affected by a larger societal issue. But in general, ethics committees try to stay focused on the many problems generated by serious illness and its medical and surgical treatment.

When one consults with an ethics committee, all the proceedings are strictly confidential. Committee members recognize the tremendous sensitivity and importance of any discussion or written communication of cases. In addition to the delicate considerations in the interplay between ethics and medicine, often there is a legal undercurrent (fear of a malpractice suit) or a threatened medical ego to deal with in a case where things have not gone just right.

So who are the people who make up an ethics committee in a typical hospital? A committee usually consists of seven to twenty-one members. Some committees are dominated by medical staff, but most attempt to carefully balance membership. There may be doctors, a lawyer, a member of the clergy, a social worker, representatives from nursing, from hospital administration, perhaps one or two representatives from the community at large, and maybe the hospital ethicist, who may or may not chair the committee. Ideally the committee should sit as a chartered, recognized hospital committee under its bylaws and procedures. To be effective, the committee must have at least the tacit approval of the three most powerful groups in the hospital body politic—namely, the medical staff, the nursing staff, and the administration.

Hospital ethics committees are excellent bodies for airing and elucidating complex issues. They also serve the crucial function of sharing the burden of decisionmaking among a community of concerned individuals. When they work well, and they don't always, hospital ethics committees can tap the wisdom of discernment of its many members. Sometimes the group wisdom can exceed the sum of its individual members.

TAPPING ETHICS RESOURCES

CHAPLAINS

Often serious illness or disability can lead to a crisis of the spirit. Likewise, a refreshment of the spirit can aid physical and emotional healing. The dynamic interplay among body, spirit, and psyche together constitute the complete entity we call a person. Twentieth-century science and the overwhelming cultural preference for the quick medical fix have reduced the patient as person to a collection of body systems in the various fields of specialty. Thus we have a doctor for the heart, one for the kidneys, and so on. Curiously, we have at least three specialists for the head: a neurosurgeon to operate on the physical structures of the brain, a neurologist for electro-control problems of the nervous system, and a psychiatrist for emotional and purely mental problems of the brain/mind. Problems of the heart, soul, and spirit are generally not considered to be in the realm of medicine, though some healers who wish to treat the whole person certainly do take these aspects of the patient into account.

Spiritual problems also fall to the specialist. Some persons of faith rely on their ongoing personal relationship with a pastor to help and guide them through the storms of illness. Others take advantage of the presence of chaplains as part of the hospital's service to the patient. The experience of chaplains in understanding the spiritual milieu of the hospital makes their services invaluable. Larger medical centers will provide a Catholic, Jewish, and Protestant chaplain who is available for informal talk or more directed spiritual counseling. In large metropolitan hospitals, ministers and leaders of other religions—Islam, Buddhism, Hinduism—are also available for patients.

Sometimes the presence of a member of the clergy or a hospital chaplain can be tremendously helpful in helping a patient make an ethical choice about their treatment. This is most true when a patient is concerned about complying with their faith's position regarding an issue. Jehovah's Witnesses are generally very conscientious about avoiding the use of blood products. However when a surgeon proposes to salvage the patient's own blood in the operating room, and reintroduce it back into the body, this procedure may motivate the Witness to seek some guidance from a local minister or teacher. Likewise a Catholic may wish a clarification of the Church's teaching regarding refusal or withdrawal of a feeding tube. I have seen many ethical impasses become unstuck with the intervention of timely advice and sympathetic support from healers of the spirit.

I would also argue that even the doubter or the unbeliever who is stuck in an ethical dilemma may find the insight of a hospital chaplain to be helpful. Perhaps even considering the multiple perspectives of many different chaplains may make a hard choice easier.

SOCIAL WORKER

Hospital social workers are very attuned to the labyrinthine structures of health care. They are trained to negotiate the social structure of the hospital as well as the complex network of offices, programs, and other resources that are available to aid patients from outside the hospital. They regularly deal with such things as arranging home health care, obtaining help for patients from the welfare system, or assisting in nursing home placements.

Should a crisis in care develop during a hospital stay, a skilled social worker can be very adept at gaining access to the right channels of aid. Social workers have a good practical sense of the realities of disease. Those who direct most of their energies to the intensive care unit are very familiar with the common pitfalls of decisionmaking in this environment. They can be extremely helpful to patients and family because of their ability to rapidly mobilize the diverse resources of the institution.

Though social workers spend a lot of time beating their fists against bureaucracy's door, they are often successful in their efforts. Though the medical system often dumps intractable problems in their laps, social workers seem to have the ability to proceed in hope. Think of them as potential allies when the choices are tough.

OMBUDSPERSON

Some of the larger medical centers have an office of the ombudsman or ombudswoman. If this person or office is properly constituted as an independent advocate for patient rights and is free of heavy-handed administrative pressures, it should be considered a possible aid in making moral decisions in the hospital.

An ombudsperson is constantly involved in the resolution of conflicts. Patients expect or desire a certain level of service, be it medical, nursing, or dietetics. Some patients are more assertive than others and will scream when they think their rights are being violated. Sometimes their rights *are* violated. Besides the common complaints about meals and billing, patients complain most often about the unnecessary irritation of "routine procedures." They object to a lack of access by visitors and being denied the right to read their own medical record. And of course there is an area of patient concern so large that I have devoted an entire chapter to it—informed consent. (See Chapter 1.)

Patients will bitterly complain to the ombudsperson when they feel they have not been adequately informed about the risks of a procedure or have been painted a too-rosy picture of the expected results of a surgery. Sometimes there is a wide variance in the surgeon's and the patient's definition of just what constitutes a success.

The office of the ombudsperson is not to be confused with a hospital's office of patient services or office of patient relations. These kinds of services also aim to rectify errors, to cut off trouble, and to answer patient complaints. But the personnel in this kind of structure serve the public-relation needs of the institution. The aim is to smooth over, apologize if necessary, and preserve the unbruised name of the medical center. As such, this kind of office has no power to independently investigate, make findings, or advocate the rights of the patient. It's the difference between having your own lawyer in a legal dispute and relying on the advice of the company lawyer.

An ombudsperson could be potentially useful in a complex set of circumstances involving troubled decisionmaking. Certainly a competent ombudsperson could contribute much in the way of fact-finding that in turn could lead to a more informed decision.

HOME HEALTH CARE

In recent years there has been a distinct trend toward providing care in the home. Patients are leaving hospitals following illness "quicker and sicker" than in the past, when hospital costs were not seen to be mounting at an exponential rate. After surgery or an acute illness nowadays it is common for the physician to coordinate specialized and skilled care in the home so as to maximize chances for rapid recovery and rehabilitation.

This kind of care is provided not only by nurses, but by respiratory and occupational therapists as well. All of these health workers are committed to the idea that the home has inherent advantages for healing. It is much easier to be relaxed among friendly faces in a familiar environment. Medical treatment carried out in the home also gives the patient the feeling of having real control over treatment decisions.

The fact that interactions with the health-care system occur on home turf can make a considerable difference in how empowered you may feel. Remember that the nurses and others who may come into your home have as a result of their experience a deep knowledge and a wide perspective about the recovery process from serious illness. So it follows that they are potential sources of information and advice about dicey care decisions that may arise.

HOSPICE

Hospice, or the expert care of the terminally ill, has grown in the last twenty years from a small movement in Great Britain to a more or less accepted, though underutilized, part of American health care. Though hospice is now reimbursed by Medicare, it is unfortunately patchy in its geographic coverage, bound by burdensome Medicare regulations, and is considered a care alternative by only a very small percentage of dying people.

Hospice emphasizes the flexible team approach to care for the dying. Typically, a doctor, a nurse, and a social worker will evaluate the patient. Of paramount importance is the alleviation of pain, which historically in the case of cancer patients has been well controlled in only about twenty-five percent of its victims. Hospice also concentrates on the emotional component of pain and suffering—the anguish of a person bound to a death-dealing disease.

Hospice now has over 1,700 independent chapters in the United States. They are organized as home-centered (most), hospital-based (some), and free-standing institutions (few). As the percentage of Americans who die in hospitals and nursing homes continues to rise, hospice will become increasingly well known as an alternative that offers more options and more control for dying persons.

My experience has been that even when critically ill patients and their family realize that a cure is not possible and that the life that is left is not long, they seem to be mired in the hospital culture. They hate the hospital and yet they don't seem to be able to leave. Even those patients who have heard of hospice and want it for themselves often wait too long to avail themselves of a more comforting way of dying.

Hospice will accept patients who are expected to live for six or fewer months. Nurses and social workers are almost always aware of this community resource. Talking to a hospice representative when in the hospital can begin to answer questions to see if hospice can serve the needs of a particular patient. Since family involvement is fundamental to the hospice philosophy, the earlier that relatives can participate in hospice planning, the better for the patient. Given their closeness to the dying, hospice workers develop a commitment as well as an ease in dealing with values in end-of-life issues. They are an excellent source of information and advice.

LAWYERS

Lawyers are primed to think about worst-case scenarios. They have the ability to predict outcomes and devise strategies to counter or cushion detrimental happenings. This is why a personal attorney might be an ideal adviser in planning a living will or a durable power or attorney instrument.

A lawyer may be a good counselor if a hospital or doctor is recalcitrant in providing the kind of care a patient wishes. For example, a patient and family may decide to forgo the insertion of a feeding tube, but the doctors in the case dig in their heels and threaten to obtain a court order for the tube. This is an area of controversy where bioethics and the law come together. Since the law is rapidly evolving in cases of hydration and nutrition, a lawyer, especially one previously known to the family, may be an ideal choice to help you work through this problem. Also, the Cruzan decision has opened the way to considerable discretion in these matters by each state. Legislation on living wills and durable powers of attorney differs from state to state. For example, New York and Missouri require a very high and specific standard of written intent for the advance directives of an incompetent patient to be given binding weight on the caregivers. There is apt to be future legislation dealing with the specific issue of artificial hydration and nutrition that will be proposed by various state legislatures. All of this present and pending legal complexity argues for professional advice when a situation develops where there is a potential legal problem arising from a patient choice in treatment decisions.

Hospitals also employ lawyers. The larger ones typically have their own legal department; the smaller health-care institutions hire legal advice on an as-needed basis. Often it is the case that physicians are both uninformed and fearful of the law pertaining to the care of patients. The hospital attorney often serves a very useful function by educating staff physicians to their obligations as well as the pitfalls of providing care. In situations where patient and family stand firmly for one option and the doctor stands on the other side of the issue, the mediating skills of an attorney can play an important role. I can recall several cases where an impasse seemed to have been reached (both parties were predicting dire legal consequences, the physician for withdrawing a respirator, the family for not withdrawing the respirator) until the hospital lawyer brought everyone up-to-date on the current legal situation.

Of course there is a danger that the very complicated issues in ethics that involve life values, personal convictions, and philosophical arguments can be oversimplified and reduced to a legal opinion. Physicians often tend to reduce bioethics to a pair of simple propositions: 1. Can I get sued for doing or not doing this or that? and 2. Is my rear covered? This kind of simplistic and self-serving ethic is inadequate to deal with the present problems that thousands of patients are facing.

A further word about hospital attorneys. Remember always, no matter how it may seem in any possible interaction with them, that they represent the interests of the medical center and none other. Their wish is to avoid conflict, minimize litigation, and solve problems on behalf of the institution. All kinds of problems come their way from the most technical to the most ridiculous. One hospital attorney I know had to legally defend his institution from the claim of a patient who accused a patient-care representative of biting his Seeing Eye dog when he left the dog in her office to go to a medical appointment. He proudly and successfully defended the hospital, but of course got into trouble with animal rights advocates. I remember him entering the cafeteria one day after the case had appeared in the newspaper greeted by a chorus of barks.

If a patient or a family acting on behalf of a patient needs an attorney for advice or to obtain redress, one must be hired. There is no substitute for independent counsel. The ideal counselor would be the attorney who knows the patient and can therefore offer informal advice based on legal and personal insights. This combination will serve the patient well in obtaining the kind and quality of health care desired. And it is the kind of advice that goes beyond mere rights, hostile confrontation, and threatened litigation.

THE MEDICAL LIBRARY

In hospitals of any size there is surely a medical library established for the medical, nursing, and allied health staffs as well as for residents (doctors in training) in the hospital. The library is a resource necessary to the professional in order to do research and to keep current in developments in health care. Often the medical library is hidden away in an old wing of the hospital or down an unpromising hallway. But if you spend much time in a hospital, as patients and their families necessarily do, you might stumble upon this place of books and journals and computer terminals. A simple inquiry to practically any hospital employee would bring you directions to the library if you were inclined to visit.

I believe you should be so inclined to seek and find this marvelous resource of medical information, knowledge, and sometimes wisdom. The first person you will encounter will be the inevitably helpful medical librarian. He or she may first think that you are after the latest fiction or mystery story, and in a way you are, but not quite how they would think. Once they know you are a serious seeker of what is referred to as the "medical literature," they will help you toward your goal.

The medical library can be helpful to patients in at least two ways. First, it can provide background information plus the latest research about a particular disease process. If one had the diagnosis of prostatic cancer, a textbook in urology or oncology would provide a chapter of medical reading on the subject—the natural history of the disease, diagnostic techniques, and standard therapies. If one consulted the *Index Medicus* for the last couple of years, the latest articles and research findings that are relevant to prostatic cancer would be listed by title, subject, and author.

The second major help for a patient enmeshed in the trial of making a difficult decision in biomedical ethics is to consult the literature that has been created, especially in the last ten years, relevant to this topic. There is a rich variety of books and articles that deal with all the issues touched upon in this book, plus many more. There are textbooks of medical ethics, there are books devoted to such issues as patient autonomy, reproductive technologies, and withholding and withdrawing treatment. There are several periodicals whose aim is to study bioethics from a multidisciplinary perspective. There are other journals whose bent is more philosophical or religious or legal. The scholarly literature in bioethics is referenced similarly to the scientific medical literature—by author, title, and subject.

Hospital medical libraries are often modest in size. Do not let these small spaces fool you. Library research in medicine has become highly computerized. Often the article or book that you may need will not be physically present in the hospital, but rather would be available on a lending basis for a book, or a copy basis for an article, from a large university collection in the region. Even the search for appropriate sources is highly computerized. The National Library of Medicine in Bethesda, Maryland, operates several computer databases including *Medline* and *Bioethics Line* which allow the user to research topics via a computer terminal. Often the hospital librarian will offer this service or at least assist in your search. The rapid access to the literature allows a comprehensive search of an ethics topic. The computer is even capable of printing abstracts of articles so that their relevance can be determined before ordering a copy of the complete article.

Another way to approach the knowledge that may inform ethical judgment is to ask your attending physician to give you a selection of articles that would be pertinent to the case at hand. True, this would be an unusual request, but it certainly tells the physician that as a patient you take more than just a passing interest in your own case. Further, it puts the physician on notice in a gentle way that you intend to know your own disease well and have a knowledge base that could question any therapeutic decision that the caregivers might make.

The hospital library might also be a source of videotapes used in ethics education for the hospital staff. There are many independent productions on ethics topics ranging from dramatizations of clinical dilemmas to discussion forums about the state of medicine and ethics. Many productions on public television are outstanding in the breadth, depth, and clarity of presentation. Only public stations would, for example, telecast Frederick Wiseman's six-hour documentary film *Near Death*. This film shows the inner workings of an intensive care unit at Beth Israel Hospital in Boston and illustrates the complex dynamics among three patients, their families, and the medical and nursing team.

What follows is a compendium of resources that may assist you to reflect more broadly and deeply about issues in bioethics. This is by no means an exhaustive list, but, rather, a rich place to begin. My experience is that one good source leads to another, then quite unexpectedly to a third, and so on. The literature grows daily—both scholarly material and works meant for a wider audience.

Five books to begin with:

The Nichomachean Ethics by Aristotle

What Kind of Life: The Limits of Medical Progress by Daniel Callahan (New York: Simon and Schuster, 1990)

Toward a More Natural Science: Biology and Human Affairs by Leon R. Kass (New York: Free Press, 1985)

The Rights of Patients: the Basic ACLU Guide to Patient Rights by George Annas, 2nd rev. ed. (Totowa, NJ: The Humana Press, 1992)

The Silent World of Doctor and Patient by Jay Katz (New York: Free Press, 1984)

Some additional distinguished writers and thinkers in bioethics:
Howard Brody, Daniel Callahan, Alexander Capron, James Childress, Larry Churchill, Albert Jonsen, Ruth Macklin, Mary Mahowald, William May, Thomas Murray, Edmund Pellegrino, Stephen Post, Paul Ramsey, and Warren Reich

Periodicals:

The Hastings Center Report
Journal of the American Medical Association
The New England Journal of Medicine
Journal of Clinical Ethics
Journal of Theoretical Medicine
Soundings
Literature and Medicine
Journal of Medical Ethics
Medical Humanities Review
Law, Medicine and Health Care
American Journal of Law & Medicine
Journal of Medical Humanities

TAPPING ETHICS RESOURCES

Films:

Near Death directed by Frederick Wiseman, 1989

Crimes and Misdemeanors directed by Woody Allen, 1989

Johnny Got His Gun directed by Dalton Trumbo, 1971

Stories, Essays, Poems:

The Death of Ivan Ilyich by Leo Tolstoy

Letters to a Young Doctor by Richard Selzer

Healing the Wounds by David Hilfiker

Awakenings by Oliver Sacks

The Doctor Stories by William Carlos Williams

Full Measure: Modern Short Stories about Aging edited by Dorothy Sennett

On Doctoring edited by Richard Reynolds and John Stone

Vital Lines: Contemporary Fiction about Medicine edited by Jon Mukand

Sutured Words: Contemporary Poetry about Medicine edited by Jon Mukand

Bioethics documents:

The Hippocratic Oath

A Patient's Bill of Rights (American Hospital Association)

Guidelines on the Termination of Life-sustaining Treatment and the Care of the Dying (The Hastings Center)

Organizations:

The Hastings Center
255 Elm Road
Briarcliff Manor, NY 10510
(914) 762-8500

American Society of Law and Medicine
765 Commonwealth Avenue
Boston, MA 02215
(617) 262-4990

Choice in Dying
200 Varick Street
New York, NY 10014
(212) 366-5540

The National Hospice Organization
1901 North Ft. Myer Drive
Suite 902
Arlington, VA 22209
(703) 243-5900

People's Medical Society
14 East Minor St.
Emmaus, PA 18049
(215) 967-2136

Society for Bioethics Consultation
c/o The Office of Bioethics
The Cleveland Clinic Foundation
9500 Euclid Avenue
Cleveland, OH 44195
(216) 444-8720

TAPPING ETHICS RESOURCES

The Park Ridge Center
1875 Dempster Street
Suite 175
Park Ridge, IL 60068
(708) 696-6399

Office of Bioethics
The Cleveland Clinic Foundation
9500 Euclid Avenue
Cleveland, OH 44195
(216) 444-8720

Institute for Medical Humanities
University of Texas Medical Branch
Galveston, TX 77550
(409) 772-2376

Midwest Bioethics Center
410 Archibald, Suite 106
Kansas City, MO 64111
(816) 756-2713

Center for Medical Ethics
University of Pittsburgh
167 Lothrup Hall
190 Lothrup Street
Pittsburgh, PA 15261
(412) 648-2150

Public Citizen Health Research Group
2000 P St. NW
Suite 708
Washington, DC 20036
(202) 872-0320

Society for Health and Human Values
6728 Old McLean Village Drive
McLean, VA 22101
(703) 556-9222

Center for Clinical Medical Ethics
University of Chicago
Box 72
5841 S. Maryland Avenue
Chicago, IL 60637
(312) 702-1453

Center for Biomedical Ethics
Case Western Reserve University School of Medicine
2109 Adelbert Road
Cleveland, OH 44106
(216) 368-6205

Institute for Humanities and Medicine
Northeastern Ohio Universities College of Medicine
P.O. Box 95
Rootstown, OH 44272
(216) 325-2511

Center for Ethics and Humanities in the Life Sciences
Michigan State University
East Lansing, MI 48821
(517) 355-7550

Kennedy Center for Ethics
Georgetown University
Washington, DC 20007
(202) 687-6774

TAPPING ETHICS RESOURCES

Center for Ethics, Medicine and Public Issues
Baylor College of Medicine
One Baylor Plaza
Houston, TX 77030
(713) 798-6290

The Program in Ethics and the Professions
Harvard University
79 Kennedy St.
Cambridge, MA 02138
(617) 495-9386

Department of Ethics and Medical History
SB-20 University of Washington
Seattle, WA 98195
(206) 543-5447

Program for Ethics and Human Values
Northwestern University Medical School
303 E. Chicago Ave.
Chicago, IL 60611
(312) 503-7962

Institute of Medicine and Humanities
P.O. Box 4587
Missoula, MT 59806
(406) 543-7271

Center for Biomedical Ethics
University of Minnesota
Minneapolis, MN 55455
(612) 625-4917

Postscript

I am reminded that the notion of choice tends to be framed in the personal sense. But there is also a community sense of choice in health-care decisions. And it seems to me the underlying problem facing the American community of caregivers and patients (and remember we all at one time or another are patients) is access to the medical system. This book can be helpful only to the person who has been able to enter the care system. In the United States in the last decade of the twentieth century over thirty-seven million of our fellow citizens do not have health care insurance. This effectively deals them out of the community of the sick, except on an emergency or charity basis. Millions more find themselves without medical insurance when they change jobs or become unemployed.

This means that we have an unjust method of delivering health care. It means that we effectively disguise the rationing of health care by allowing people into the system based often on economic means. As a physician, I daily see patients whose principal concern about their visit is how they can manage to pay for it. I recently saw a thirty-one-year-old man who was having a problem with migraine headaches. In the course of his physical exam I noted that his right cornea was clouded over. He said he was blind in that eye. He said an operation on his retina could probably restore his vision. He had no money for such a surgery, no health-care insurance, and was not poor enough to qualify for Medicaid. His plight brought to mind conversations I have had with other physicians about the Canadian health system (In Canada, all citizens have equal benefits in a one-payer system) where, according to my colleagues, one had to wait in line for weeks or months for elective surgery. And here before me was this man with no line even to stand in.

As a physician, an American, a human being, I am embarrassed and dismayed by the blatant violations of simple justice that are so common to our widely heralded practice of medicine. So I feel all the talk in this book about care choices would ring somewhat hollow to any person barred from care. Much groundwork needs to be done at the political and social level to create equal access to a basic package of health benefits for all citizens. Until that is accomplished, the ethical foundation that undergirds the entire enterprise of U.S. medicine is on shaky ground indeed.

As a community, we have a collective choice that will define the heart of the kind of care system we want. Will health care be based on excluding the poor, the jobless, the unfortunate, or will the American community of caring strive to include everyone?

APPENDIX I

The Technology of Intensive Care

The Technology Train

Nowhere in the hospital is the crunch of technology and ethics more troublesome than in the intensive care unit. For it is there that medicine's latest and finest devices and techniques to measure, monitor, and treat have outrun the human need to ponder, reflect, and make informed decisions. The fast train of technology makes no stops. Indeed, the passengers sense that the train is continually accelerating. One is left with the impression that thinking about the meaning of things is a concept that has been left back at the station. Aristotle and his ilk are but a dim memory and have been left a long way back in time. The technological imperative—what can be done will be done—has its hand on the throttle. The tracks stretch out into the distance. Parallel lines converge in the fog. The whistle blows. Is anyone out there listening?

Intensive care units treat life-threatening illnesses and injuries. They are staffed with highly trained nurses and doctors and other health workers such as respiratory therapists, who have a range of highly sophisticated equipment at their disposal. The different names of intensive care units show the specialization of their task: neonatal intensive care unit (NICU); medical intensive care unit (MICU); surgical intensive care unit (SICU); and so on. The patients in these various units are at the very least seriously ill. Many are critically ill, some gravely ill.

The Place of Critical-Care Medicine

The last twenty years of American medicine has seen intensive care proliferate. There are over sixty thousand intensive care beds in U.S. hospitals accounting for ten percent of our total health bill, over sixty billion dollars a year. The average daily cost to the patient is something on the order of two thousand dollars per day. Although insurance companies (third-party payers) and government-entitlement programs pick up the tab for most people, in the end, one way or another, through taxes or premiums, we all pay. Death itself has become institutionalized. Whereas in 1949, fifty percent of Americans died at home, by 1980 fully eighty percent were spending their last days in a hospital or nursing home.

Family members who go to an intensive care unit for the first time to visit a relative are often shocked at the scene before them. There in a cubicle perhaps eight feet by ten feet is a bed surrounded by all manner of instrumentation and strange-looking devices. In the bed their loved one is attached to numerous tubes, seemingly in every bodily orifice, and more. Simple things like talking and touching are significantly impeded in the "unit." The sounds of electronic monitors and alarms and telephones and beepers create an orchestra of dissonance. Nurses, residents, ward clerks, and technicians create a bustle of never-ending busyness. To say the least, the scene is intimidating to anyone unaccustomed to such a world. One of the aims of this appendix is to demystify the intensive care unit.

The need to understand the function and implications of intensive-care medicine is underscored by the sheer numbers of Americans who have had firsthand experience with this most imposing place of care. One recent poll of over one thousand adult Texans reported that over fifty percent of the people had faced a life and death decision in their family in the previous two years. Often the serious illness of a parent unites a family in the ICU waiting room for long, grim hours. These family members get to see high-tech medicine up close and are often surprised at how very close to their hometowns the future has come.

Technology and Choices

Making decisions in medicine is often difficult under the best of circumstances. The intense, dangerous, alienating, otherworldly aspects of the ICU multiply the stress both on caregivers and family members. To know this world better will not only alleviate some degree of stress, but will enable the choices of care to be better understood.

The first task in considering care is to learn just what the possibilities are from a medical technology point of view. To understand the menu of options requires a grounding in the available medical hardware and techniques. Only when the purely medical considerations are thoroughly understood can the larger questions of the appropriateness of treatment be entertained. Because there is a human center in medicine, the human dimension should suffuse the entire enterprise of care. Since a patient is not merely a collection of biological systems, the ethical questions about care move to the forefront. As illness magnifies human vulnerability, and as technology in turn blurs human features, great care must be exercised in recognizing and protecting the core integrity of the person bound by the wires, tubes, and machines of the intensive care unit.

Agnes and Virgil

Sometimes a patient loses his identity in the ICU. The story of Agnes and Virgil Tompkins is instructive. Virgil is a fifty-six-year-old electrician in a small town in northern Ohio. For a time last year he suffered from intense headaches that came on suddenly, blurring his vision and "making my head feel like someone was shoving a red-hot ice pick into my left temple," he explained to his doctor. In fact, the pain was so bad he could not work, nor could he hide it from Agnes. She could tell by the look of helplessness and befuddlement in his eyes that something serious was going on. The CAT scan in Toledo showed a brain tumor and soon Virgil was scheduled for surgery. The surgery went well and a large, nonmalignant growth was removed from his brain.

Agnes Tompkins paced and worried in the surgery waiting room. When the neurosurgeon came down and told her that everything had gone well, she sighed a great sigh and asked if she could see her husband later that evening when he was transferred from the surgical recovery room to the neurological intensive care unit. The doctor agreed that would be a great idea and would lift Virgil's spirits. So Agnes went up to the ICU during visiting hours about an hour and a half after talking to his surgeon. She looked for cubicle number 14, where she saw her be-tubed and bandaged husband. She held his hand and repeated the good news she had heard from his doctor. He just moaned in response, not even opening his eyes. He could not have spoken even if he wanted to, since he had a breathing tube down his throat. Agnes spoke soothingly and was glad to be in the same room with him.

After about ten minutes she went over to the nurses' desk to ask about her husband's grogginess. A nurse looked at her visitor's name badge and told her that they would be bringing her husband up to cubicle 4 within half an hour. Agnes Tompkins swallowed hard, let out only a high-pitched peep in her effort to speak, then recovered, saying that her husband was in number 14. Oh, no, they assured her, that's Mr. Solinski. He's been here since midafternoon. That's Mr. Solinski, sorry.

Well, Virgil and Agnes eventually both recovered. And now Agnes pays special attention to her husband's work-roughened hands.

The audience for this book is the patient in that ICU cubicle. This person is potentially me, and, of course, it could be you. The audience is also the family gathered together in the waiting room, waiting for the drama of husband or grandfather to play out, hoping for deliverance from a fate seemingly bound to the creations of engineers and scientists, seeking solace and also the wisdom that they may with their loved one do the right thing.

ICU Technology: Procedures and Devices

CPR

The first technical treatment to consider is cardiopulmonary resuscitation, better known as CPR. This potentially lifesaving technique involves artificially sustaining and attempting to restart the heart-lung systems that have stopped (either alone or in tandem). This is a situation known as cardiac arrest or respiratory arrest or cardiopulmonary arrest. This circumstance precipitates a "code," that is a rapid, coordinated response from nearby health workers followed soon by a special code team that takes over the administration of CPR. The team is headed by a physician skilled in the technique of resuscitation.

The first action taken often consists of a hard, sharp blow to the chest with a fist. Sometimes this "precordial thump" will by itself restore the heart to a normal rhythm. But in most cases cardiopulmonary resuscitation must begin. CPR consists of chest compressions to move blood through the circulatory system by in effect squeezing the heart from the outside. At the same time, it is necessary to breathe for the patient. This is done initially by forcing air into the lungs via a mouthpiece or a hand-held breathing bag. Respirations are then timed with chest compressions so that oxygen can get into the lungs, where it is exchanged with the carbon dioxide being released from the bloodstream. Sometimes the chest compressions cause bruising and even fractured ribs due to the vigorous nature of the technique and the brittle consistency of some older bones.

When the code team arrives, the patient is immediately intubated. Intubation is the passing of a soft plastic tube about the diameter of your pinky down the throat and into the windpipe.

The tube can then be hooked up to an oxygen supply along with a breathing bag (if this device is not already in use), thereby establishing a very effective and potentially lifesaving airway.

The team then attempts to stimulate the heart back to functioning as an efficient blood pump. This is done through potent stimulating drugs administered directly into the bloodstream or sometimes by direct injection with a long needle into the heart muscle itself. Other drugs are given in order to retain or regain a steady, regular heartbeat. During the entire code the heart is electronically monitored so that the clinicians can determine the exact kind of heart problem that is occurring.

The last technique at the disposal of the resuscitation team is the application of an electric charge or shock to the heart muscle. This is done in order to effect a change in a heart rate or rhythm that is harmful to the patient. By dramatically applying an electric shock to the chest wall, chaotic rhythms are abolished as the built-in pathways of nerve transmission are often shocked back to a normal, life-sustaining rhythm. This process is sometimes termed "defibrillation," since when the heart beats wildly and ineffectively it is said to be fibrillating. The device used to restore normal cardiac rhythm is called a defibrillator.

INTRAVENOUS LINES (IVS)

"Doc, don't let them hook me up to all those tubes." I think every physician at one time or another has heard this remark. Tubes that penetrate the body do have a somewhat frightening prospect about them. In a real and palpable way they are an invasion of bodily integrity and, like all technology, represent a blurring of the body's boundaries.

Intravenous access, or IVs, have been commonly used in medicine since the 1930s, following early and dangerous experiments in the seventeenth century by Christopher Wren and later in 1851 by Charles Gabriel Pravaz, who invented the hypodermic needle. They are of two general types—peripheral and central intravenous lines. IVs are generally started in the arm and are used for giving fluids and medications. Fluids are often needed by ill or injured persons to replace losses in the course of a medical illness or an injury such as a burn. Likewise, a person unable to take in or tolerate an oral fluid intake, perhaps because of nausea and vomiting, or, more seriously, because of impairment from a stroke, can be helped with IV fluid therapy. The right mix of water, salt, sugar, and minerals, administered through an IV, can keep a patient balanced with respect to the body's fluid needs.

A central IV can be thought of as a large-caliber tube that is generally threaded into a large vein in the neck or just above the collarbone. This kind of venous access allows large volumes of replacement fluids or medication to be administered quickly. It also provides an access for a thicker, more nutritious fluid to be supplied to the patient who is unable to eat. This feeding technique, called TPN, will be discussed later in this appendix.

BLOOD

Intravenous lines provide the portal for blood and blood products to enter the body. Transfusions of matched whole blood or blood cells or certain factors derived from blood can be lifesaving for the patient who has bled, either slowly and chronically or acutely, as after an automobile accident. Blood products are the separated and purified specific elements of whole blood that are used to treat everything from hemophilia (factor VIII) to clotting deficiencies (platelets). Blood and blood products should be seen as valuable resources used in the care of seriously ill patients who do not object on religious grounds.

Scrupulous screening of donated blood cannot prevent the transmission of some forms of hepatitis, a viral liver infection, in from three to ten percent of blood-product recipients. The risk increases as the number of transfusions increases. To avoid this risk, it is sometimes possible to plan ahead and donate blood to yourself (autologous transfusion). This blood is collected and then banked until such time that it might be needed for an elective surgery. Needless to say, this kind of preparation is not always possible, as in the event of an emergency or in the case of a person too weak and chronically ill to donate blood.

VASOPRESSORS

Vasopressors are a category of drug often used in the ICU setting. These potent agents stimulate the heart to beat more efficiently and with greater force. This category of drug also stimulates the muscle tissue within the walls of arteries to contract. This clamping-down effect diminishes the diameter of the blood vessel. In turn, this can raise the blood pressure of the critically ill patient whose circulatory system has been compromised. Drugs like dopamine and dobutamine are usually administered by infusion or slow drip into a vein because they are effective in very small amounts and must be carefully monitored.

RESPIRATOR

A respirator is basically a breathing machine. Also called a ventilator or a vent, the device inflates and deflates the lungs. Typically, the respirator is used during surgery, when a body's systems are under the mechanical and pharmacological control of

THE TECHNOLOGY OF INTENSIVE CARE

the anesthesiologist. The trachea, or windpipe, is first intubated with a pliable, firm plastic tube which is then hooked up to the respirator.

The respirator supplies the lungs with a steady supply of air at a breathing rate determined by the doctor. The percentage of oxygen and anesthetic inhalants in the mixture is also precisely regulated during and after surgery. In the recovery room following surgery, the patient is taken off the ventilator, if possible, before being sent to an intensive care unit for recovery.

Heart failure, respiratory distress syndrome, and illnesses such as severe asthma often require that the patient be put on a respirator in order to properly nourish the body's cells with enough oxygen. Seriously ill patients, especially the elderly, are sometimes so weakened from the process of a disease that they are unable to breathe without mechanical support. Most intensive-care patients are respirator dependent for the time of the acute phase of their illness. Then the physician and respiratory therapist will attempt to wean the patient from their dependence on the respirator. This is often not easily accomplished in older, more debilitated patients and sometimes takes some weeks to accomplish completely. This is often due to the atrophied or weakened state of the breathing muscles, such as the diaphragm, that have shrunk through lack of use. In some unfortunate cases, weaning from the ventilator is impossible.

Being confined to an ICU cubicle for a long period of time is very isolating and alienating even without considering the added burden of a respirator. The loss of time orientation, the deprivation of the natural patterns of day and night, the surreal sight and sound of machines, the constant change of staff, the pain, the anxiety, the interrupted sleep, all contribute to an entity known as ICU psychosis. The patient may become combative, be depressed, or entertain hallucinations. Add to this series of physical and psychological insults of a breathing tube that makes speech impossible, and you have a prescription for personal terror.

DIALYSIS

Kidneys filter the blood, taking out toxins and unneeded residues and dumping them into the bladder, where the body stores and eliminates the liquid waste. Sometimes in acute illness or as a result of a long-term illness like diabetes, the kidneys will stop working. Other times a particular affliction of the kidneys themselves, such as drug poisoning, infection, or inflammation will cause the kidneys to stop functioning. Since the heart, lungs, and kidneys are interdependent, as are the other organ systems, a disease that affects one organ can affect others. For example, in heart failure, the inefficient pumping of blood by the heart muscle and the sluggish flow of blood may cause the kidneys to suffer as well. In this case, treating the underlying heart problem will tend to solve the insufficient flow of blood to the kidney.

Kidney failure may be temporary or permanent. It may result from a chronic illness or from an acute insult. The kidney dialysis machine is a complex artificial filtering device that can be hooked up to a patient for periodic cleansing of the blood. The interval between dialysis treatment varies, but is usually three times a week.

In the hospital, hemodialysis is accomplished by accessing the patient's veins, running the blood at a controlled rate through the machine, and returning the blood to the circulatory system. Another form of outpatient dialysis called chronic ambulatory peritoneal dialysis (CAPD), is not generally used in acute situations.

Since the decision to go on dialysis may be lifesaving, it is yet another critical decision to be made in the ICU. Like other technically sophisticated therapies, dialysis has both burdens and benefits. Long-term dialysis patients have an extremely high suicide rate. Many other patients eventually decide to forgo further treatment on the artificial kidney because of what they see as a markedly diminished quality of life due to the required strict diet and constant attention to medications and treatment regimens.

INTRA-AORTIC BALLOON PUMP

Intra-aortic balloon counterpulsation is a technique designed to assist the pumping function of a weak or damaged heart. The pump provides temporary stabilization only and cannot be used on a long-term basis.

To help the circulation, the physician enters an artery in the groin and passes a catheter up into the aorta in the chest region. The aorta, being the principal artery coming from the heart, is the Amazon of blood vessels. From this main artery flow the branches that nourish the brain, the liver, the kidneys, and the extremities. A balloon at the end of the catheter can inflate and deflate. The pump times this inflation and deflation with the regular opening and closing of the heart valves so that heart muscle and balloon together work in harmony to more efficiently pump blood.

Besides being a temporizing measure, the intra-aortic balloon pump can cause serious side effects, including perforation of a blood vessel, clots breaking loose in the circulation, decreased blood flow to legs, and possible infection at the puncture site in the groin.

CARDIAC PACEMAKER

A cardiac pacemaker consists of a power source and "brain" connected to a wire that is surgically implanted in the wall of the heart. This device paces the beating of the heart when the intrinsic electrical system of the heart malfunctions. The heart, like other electromechanical pumps, depends upon electricity for control functions. The loss of control is evident when the heart beats too slowly and thereby cannot supply the body with enough blood. This typically happens when the heart rate falls below fifty beats per minute. When this occurs, the programmed pacemaker kicks in and takes over the stimulation of the heart's rhythm.

The miniature battery pack and pacing brain are implanted beneath the skin on the chest. Occasionally a pacemaker has to be replaced or serviced and this, of course, can lead to some discomfort.

ANTIBIOTIC THERAPY

Antibiotic drug therapy to fight infection is seemingly out of place on this list of ICU technologies. After all, antibiotics are routinely given for everything from strep throat to athlete's foot. In the context of the intensive care unit, however, powerful and sophisticated antibiotic drugs are given via IVs to fight common and deadly serious hospital infections in patients who are weakened by surgery or debilitated by a long illness. The bad bugs simply spot an opportunity and move into hosts who are unprepared to effectively fight them off. Infection of the lungs is one such infection. In the old days, clinicians would often refer to pneumonia as the old person's friend—lung infections with no available antibiotic to use would lead to a rapid demise of such a patient.

Employing antibiotics in situations where they would prolong dying would be clearly inappropriate. So this kind of pharmaceutical therapy may be looked upon as yet another optional technology of the ICU.

ARTIFICIAL NUTRITION

Like other organ systems under the stress of protracted illness or acute trauma, the gastrointestinal system, too, suffers from breakdown or shutdown. Following surgery, a major burn, or a long bout with heart disease or cancer, the patient is often unable to take in anything by mouth. Peripheral IVs can supply a sugar, salt, and water solution that when properly monitored and regulated can keep a patient's fluid level in balance. But proper nutrition is another story, especially when you realize that the body needs markedly more calories when it is undergoing the tremendous stress of mobilizing itself to fight an illness or attempting to repair damaged organ systems.

The health-care team will often consult a dietician to consider the best means of feeding the ICU patient. Basically there are three choices for artificial feeding. I use the term "artificial" intentionally. Just as the respirator artificially breathes for the patient, and the dialysis machine functions as an artificial kidney, so does the technology and techniques I am about to describe artificially provide nutrition to the person whose GI tract is somehow impaired or diseased. If oral intake is impaired for a patient and the processes we take for granted—chewing, swallowing, digestion—are interrupted, then medical intervention is necessary to sustain nutrition.

The three artificial feeding techniques are nasogastric tube, gastrostomy or jejunostomy tube, and total parenteral nutrition.

The nasogastric tube is a small-caliber tube that is passed through the nose, down the throat, and into the stomach. Feeding solutions, often high in protein, are forced through the tube and into the stomach. Many patients find this type of feeding to be highly irritating and objectionable, more so after a period of time passes and the tube rubs nasal passages raw.

Gastrostomy and jejunostomy tubes are larger-caliber tubes that provide direct access to the stomach and the first part of the small intestine, respectively, without going through the mouth and throat. However, to insert the tube into the patient requires a surgical procedure in the operating room with a general anesthetic in which the surgeon essentially makes a hole in the abdominal wall and GI tract and then places a tube into the stomach or small intestine. Feedings are accomplished by blending food to a baby-food consistency or by pouring in prepared nutritional mixtures.

The third approach to feeding the patient unable to take in food by mouth is termed TPN, or total parenteral nutrition. This technique has been refined over the last twenty years so that elemental constituents of nutrition—proteins, carbohydrates, and fats—can be directly instilled into the bloodstream. The trip down a damaged alimentary canal is thereby avoided, as is the necessity for digestion. TPN requires the insertion of a large catheter into a large vein just below the right collarbone. The catheter is then sewn into place and the system is ready for the instilling of special, very sophisticated and expensive solutions, much more watery than tube-feeding mixtures. TPN must be very carefully monitored to avoid metabolic imbalances, especially blood sugar problems. Since the technique uses a direct access to the bloodstream, the risk of serious blood infection is a real consideration in choosing this type of artificial feeding.

THE TECHNOLOGY OF INTENSIVE CARE

FOLEY CATHETER

The last tube to consider in the ICU is often the first tube to be placed. This is the Foley catheter. This tube is passed through the urethra into the bladder in order to provide continuous drainage of urine by gravity feed to a plastic bag at the side of the bed. Urine output, an important thing to know about a seriously ill patient, can then be readily measured. The catheter is anchored in place by inflating a small balloon to act as a collar inside the bladder in order to thwart the intentional or inadvertent removal of the catheter.

Foley catheters, or simply "foleys," make the necessary elimination of liquid waste in the very sick patient very convenient. Their chief risk to the patient is the directly accessible communication between the outside world of bacteria and the inside of the body. Within weeks practically all hospital patients with a catheter become infected. Though most often easily treated, urinary tract infections can sometimes be not only uncomfortable to the patient but a hard-to-treat, serious infection when caused by resistant strains of organisms that proliferate in hospitals.

A more permanent solution in the chronically incontinent patient is the suprapubic catheter. This is a surgically implanted tube that goes through the abdominal wall and into the bladder. The risks of infection in this system are somewhat less because of less frequent open communication with the world of infectious agents.

RARE AND RADICAL TECHNOLOGIES

Very few ICU patients at present have to face the possibility of the so-called "cutting edge" technologies. Only the most dire of circumstances and the grimmest prognosis would occasion consideration of the following procedures:

Left Ventricular Assist Device

This is an assist pump for the major pumping chamber of the heart designed to increase the heart's output. This surgical technology is used to buy time for a cardiac transplant and is considered a "bridge" to this more definitive procedure.

Solid-Organ Transplantation

In 1988 in the United States there were 1,647 cardiac transplants, 31 lung transplants, 74 combined heart and lung transplants, 1,680 liver transplants, 243 pancreas transplants, and 9,123 kidney transplants. Except for the kidney transplants, which have been performed for years as an alternative treatment to dialysis for end-stage renal disease, the other solid-organ transplants are relatively new, massively expensive, highly risky, and enormously complex procedures that are undertaken only in selected patients (generally younger, otherwise healthy patients) who have experienced focal organ failure. Transplants raise significant social, economic, and long-term-care issues. Recipients must go on a lifelong regimen of powerful drugs that suppress the body's defense system. From a societal point of view, given that major organs eventually fail in most people and the cost of each procedure is in excess of $100,000, any decision to commit to organ transplantation on a large scale as standard treatment has the potential to literally bankrupt the health-care system.

Total Artificial Heart

This experimental surgical procedure is familiar to most Americans because of the intense media coverage of Dr. William DeVries' implantation of a mechanical pump into the chest of Barney Clark in 1982. This experimental therapy with the Jarvik 7 artificial heart was repeated in two other patients. No one survived the surgery for any length of time or with any quality of life. Clotting complications as well as the unwieldy external drive mechanism spelled an end to this particular chapter in American medicine.

Development work continues at several research centers on a totally implantable artificial heart that would be much smaller than past systems with its own power source to run an efficient mechanical pump.

Common ICU Procedures

THE HEART

EKG

The electrical activity of the heart is constantly monitored by the EKG or ECG, that is, the electrocardiogram machine. Electrodes are attached to the patient's body and the monitors are both above the bed and at the nurses' station.

CVP Line

This intravenous line goes from the neck or upper chest to just outside the right heart chamber and measures the fluid pressure of the blood returning from the circulation back to the heart.

This measure of the body's blood return is called the central venous pressure and is important for making sure the body fluids are in balance.

Swan-Ganz Catheter

This is another intravenous measuring device designed to tell the care team about the dynamics of blood flow and hence the efficiency of the heart pump. Among other measurements, this catheter determines cardiac output and the blood pressure in the vessels near the heart during the pump and rest stages of the heartbeat cycle.

LUNGS

Bronchoscopy

This procedure uses a flexible tube with a tiny light and instruments at its tip in order to probe and sample the bronchial tree for signs of disease. Often the procedure is uncomfortable, but it generally produces a definitive diagnosis.

Tracheostomy

This surgical procedure allows the breathing tube to be removed from the throat and upper windpipe of the ventilator-dependent patient. Making an incision on the front of the neck into the windpipe permits the respirator tube to be more comfortably placed. This operation is usually considered when a patient has been on the respirator for two weeks or more and has no short-term prospect of getting off.

APPENDIX II

Designation of Patient Advocate Form

And Directions for Health Care

Durable Power of Attorney for Health Care

This is an important legal document. You should discuss it with your doctor and attorney if you have questions.

To my Family, Doctors and All Concerned with my care:

These instructions express my wishes about my health care. I want my family, doctors, and everyone else concerned with my care to act in accord with them.

Appointment of Patient Advocate

I appoint the following person my Patient Advocate:

Patient Advocate's Name _____
type or print

Address _____

Appointment of Successor Patient Advocate(s)

I appoint the following person(s), in the order listed, my successor Patient Advocate if my Patient Advocate does not accept my appointment, is incapacitated, resigns or is removed. My successor Patient Advocate is to have the same powers and rights as my Patient Advocate.

Name _____
type or print
Address _____

Name _____
type or print
Address _____

Consult this column for guidance.▼

Here you name someone to act for you regarding your care, custody and treatment. This person is called a "Patient Advocate." You may name anyone who is at least eighteen years old and of sound mind. You may also name one or more persons to act if your first choice cannot.

If you change your mind, you may revoke your appointment of a Patient Advocate at any time.

My Patient Advocate or successor Patient Advocate may delegate his/her powers to the next successor Patient Advocate if he or she is unable to act.

My Patient Advocate or successor Patient Advocate may only act if I am unable to participate in making decisions regarding my medical treatment.

This section gives instructions for your care. <u>Cross out and initial</u> any instructions you do <u>not</u> want.

Under instruction 1.b., your Patient Advocate has the right to make arrangements for your care but is not required personally to pay the cost of your care.

Instructions For Care

1. GENERAL INSTRUCTIONS

My Patient Advocate shall have the authority to make all decisions and to take all actions regarding my care, custody and medical treatment including, but not limited to the following:

   a. Have access to, obtain copies of and authorize release of my medical and other personal information.

   b. Employ and discharge physicians, nurses, therapists, and any other health care providers, and arrange to pay them reasonable compensation.

   c. Consent to, refuse or withdraw for me any medical care; diagnostic, surgical, or therapeutic procedure; or other treatment of any type or nature, <u>including life-sustaining treatments</u>. I understand that life-sustaining treatment includes, but is not limited to breathing with the use of a machine and receiving food, water and other liquids through tubes. I also understand that these decisions could or would allow me to die. I have listed below any specific instructions I have related to life-sustaining treatments.

Note: Current law does not permit your Patient Advocate to make decisions to withhold or withdraw treatment if you are pregnant if that decision would result in your death, to engage in homicide or euthanasia, or to force medical treatment you do not want because of your religious beliefs.

2. SPECIFIC INSTRUCTIONS

My Patient Advocate is to be guided in making medical decisions for me by what I have told him/her about my personal preferences regarding my care. Some of my preferences are recorded below and on the following pages.

You may list specific care and treatment you do or do not want. Otherwise, your general instructions will stand for your wishes.

   a. Specific Instructions Regarding Care I Do Want.

_____
_____
_____

   b. Specific Instructions Regarding Care I Do Not Want.

_____
_____
_____

   c. Specific Instructions Regarding Life-Sustaining Treatment

      I understand that I do not have to choose one of the instructions regarding life-sustaining treatment listed below. If I choose one, I will sign below my choice.

      If I sign one of the choices listed below, I direct that reasonable measures be taken to keep me comfortable and relieve pain.

You do not have to choose one of the specific instructions about life sustaining treatment in this section. But if you do, sign only one instruction.

You should discuss these choices with your doctor.

   Choice 1: I do not want my life to be prolonged by providing or continuing life-sustaining treatment if any of the following medical conditions exist:

      I am in an irreversible coma or persistent vegetative state.

I am terminally ill and life-sustaining procedures would serve only to artificially delay my death.

Under any circumstances where my medical condition is such that the burdens of the treatment outweigh the expected benefits. In weighing the burdens and benefits of treatment, I want my Patient Advocate to consider the relief of suffering and the quality of my life as well as the extent of possibly prolonging my life.

I understand that this decision could or would allow me to die.

If this statement reflects your desires, sign here:

_____

Choice 2: I want my life to be prolonged by life-sustaining treatment <u>unless</u> I am in a coma or vegetative state which my doctor reasonably believes to be irreversible. Once my doctor has reasonably concluded that I will remain unconscious for the rest of my life, I do not want life-sustaining treatment to be provided or continued. I understand that this decision could or would allow me to die.

If this statement reflects your desires, sign here:

_____

Choice 3: I want my life to be prolonged to the greatest extent possible consistent with sound medical practice without regard to my condition, the chances I have for recovery, or the cost of my care, and I direct life-sustaining treatment be provided in order to prolong my life.

If this statement reflects your desires, sign here:

_____

d. **Specific Instructions Regarding Medical Examinations.**

My religious beliefs prohibit a medical examination to determine whether I am unable to participate in making medical treatment decision. I desire this determination to be made in the following manner:

_____
_____
_____

_____

This document is to be treated as a Durable Power of Attorney for Health Care and shall survive my disability or incapacity.

If I am unable to participate in making decisions for my care and there is no Patient Advocate or successor Patient Advocate able to act for me, I request that the instructions I have given in this document be followed and that this document be treated as conclusive evidence of my wishes.

It is also my intent that anyone participating in my medical treatment shall not be liable for following the directions in my Patient Advocate that are consistent with my instructions.

This document is signed in the State of Michigan. It is my intent that the laws of the State of Michigan govern all questions concerning its validity, the interpretation of its provisions and its enforceability. I also intent that it be applied to the fullest extent possible wherever I may be.

Photocopies of this document can be relied upon as though they were originals.

I am providing these instructions of my free will. I have not been required to give them in order to receive or have care withheld or withdrawn. I am at least eighteen years old and of sound mind.

Sign and date here <u>in the presence of at least two witnesses who meet the requirements listed in the witness statement on the following page.</u>

Signature

Sign Name _____ Date _____
Name _____
type or print
Address _____

Witness Statement And Signature

I declare that the person who signed this Designation of Patient Advocate signed it in my presence and is known to me. I also declare that the person who signed appears to be of sound mind and under no duress, fraud, or undue influence and is not my husband or wife, parent, child, grandchild, brother, or sister. I declare that I am not the presumptive heir of the person who signed the previous page, the known beneficiary of his/her will at the time of witnessing, his/her physician or a person named as the Patient Advocate. I also declare that I am not an employee of a life or health insurance provider for the person who signed, an employee of a health facility that is treating him/her, or an employee of a home for the aged where he/she resides and that I am at least eighteen years old.

Witnesses

Sign Name _____
Name _____
      type or print
Address _____
_____
Date _____

Sign Name _____
Name _____
      type or print
Address _____
_____
Date _____

Sign Name _____
Name _____
      type or print
Address _____
_____
Date _____

If the witness does not personally know the person who is signing this Designation, the witness should ask for identification, such as a driver's license.

Only two witnesses are required. Using three will protect the validity of the Designation if one witness is later found ineligible to be a witness.

Keep the signed original with your personal papers at home. Give signed copies to your doctor, family, the medical facility where you are being treated and to Patient Advocates. You should review this document from time to

REAFFIRMED

Date _____ Signature _____
Date _____ Signature _____
Date _____ Signature _____
Date _____ Signature _____
Date _____ Signature _____

time and when there is a change in your health or family status. When you review it, if it still expresses your intent, sign and date under the Reaffirmed section at right to show you still agree with its contents. If your wishes change, destroy this document, make out a new one and give a copy to everyone who has a copy of the old version.

You should discuss this document with the person you want to have as your Patient Advocate and have him/her sign the Acceptance of Patient Advocate on the next page.

Acceptance of Patient Advocate

The Patient Advocate and any successor Patient Advocate must sign this Acceptance before he/she may act as Patient Advocate.

I agree to be the Patient Advocate for _____
_____ (called "Patient" in the rest of this document). I accept the Patient's designation of me as Patient Advocate. I understand and agree to take reasonable steps to follow the desires and instructions of the Patient as indicated in the Designation of Patient Advocate, in other written instructions of the Patient and as we have discussed verbally.

I also understand and agree that:

a. This designation shall not become effective unless the Patient is unable to participate in medical treatment decisions.
b. A Patient Advocate shall not exercise powers concerning the patient's care, custody, and medical treatment that the Patient, if the Patient were able to participate in the decision, could not have exercised on his or her own behalf.
c. This designation cannot be used to make a medical treatment decision to withhold or withdraw treatment from a Patient who is pregnant that would result in the pregnant Patient's death.
d. A Patient Advocate may make a decision to withhold or withdraw treament which would allow a Patient to die only if the patient has

These restrictions are required by the Patient Advocate Act of 1990, P.A. No. 312. (MCLA 700.496)

expressed in a clear and convincing manner that the Patient Advocate is authorized to make such a decision, and that the Patient acknowledges that such a decision could or would allow the Patient's death.

e. A Patient Advocate shall not receive compensation for the performance of his or her authority, rights, and responsibilities, but a Patient Advocate may be reimbursed for actual and necessary expenses incurred in the performance of his or her authority, rights and responsibilities.

f. A Patient Advocate shall act in accordance with the standards of care applicable to fiduciaries when acting for the Patient and shall act consistent with the Patient's best interests. The known desires of the Patient expressed or evidenced while the Patient is able to participate in medical treatment decisions are presumed in the Patient's best interests.

g. A Patient may revoke his or her designation at any time and in any manner sufficient to communicate an intent to revoke.

h. A Patient Advocate may revoke his or her acceptance to the designation at any time and in any manner sufficient to communicate an intent to revoke.

i. A Patient admitted to a health facility or agency has the rights enumerated in Section 20201 of the Public Health Code, Act No. 368 of the Public Acts of 1978, being Section 333.20201 of the Michigan Compiled Laws.

Continued on following page.

If I am unavailable to act after reasonable effort to contact me, I delegate my authority to the persons the Patient has designated as successor Patient Advocate in the order designated. The successor Patient

Advocate is authorized to act until I become available to act.

This Form Approved By:

PATIENT ADVOCATE

Sign Name _____
Name _____
        type or print
Address _____
_____
Home Phone _____ Work Phone _____

Successor PATIENT ADVOCATE

Sign Name _____
Name _____
        type or print
Address _____
_____
Home Phone _____ Work Phone _____

Successor PATIENT ADVOCATE

Sign Name _____
Name _____
        type or print
Address _____
_____
Home Phone _____ Work Phone _____

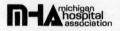

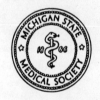

April 1991

For information about obtaining copies of the above form, write:

>Patient Advocate
>P.O. Box 950
>East Lansing, MI 48826